SAVE
YOURSELF
SOME
THERAPY

"I was blown away. Although I assumed I did not struggle with many of these areas, the more I read, the more I realized I'm bogged down by most of what Amber highlighted. The practical steps are excellent, and the discussion questions are exactly what I would expect from a seasoned counselor. I think this book will do exactly what it is intended to do."

—Natalie Nolt
Small Business Owner

"I thought it was a highly practical book and easy to read while still being thought-provoking. It had great content without being too heady, which is important for a reader who might be in a season of overwhelm. I appreciated the sense of humor—the way Amber sprinkled the book with lightheartedness was disarming and welcome after all the times she stepped on my toes."

—Trina Yoder
Small Business Owner

"All of the points Amber made about safeguarding our minds from too much stimulation pretty much floored me. Her viewpoint gave me a lot more grounding and ownership over this issue. She spoke about it so firmly and yet with so much compassion. There are tools for me!"

—Mary Campbell Norman
Educator

"The four dangers Amber lays out are huge pieces of the most common struggles I see. It is an easy read, and Amber's voice and humor make it an enjoyable one, too. I found myself underlining certain sentences to hold onto. In the margin by the quote, 'How much of our mental and emotional distress is related to our actual lives,' I wrote, 'boom.' So, so good."

Licensed Professional Counselor

"Honestly, the only thing I would change is dialing up the 'promise' in the introduction. To me, this book—if read and applied—really would 'save people some therapy,' which makes me think Amber could promise *more* of that in the introduction. I think it would be tough to *overpromise* the helpfulness of this book."

—**Kent Bateman**
Pastor

"I really enjoyed reading this book! Amber has a gift to communicate big ideas in understandable and livable ways."

—**Peter Hubbard**
Pastor and Author of *Love Into Light*

Four Modern Dangers to Our Mental Health
and What to Do About It

SAVE YOURSELF SOME THERAPY

AMBER BATEMAN, LPC

Ambassador International
GREENVILLE, SOUTH CAROLINA & BELFAST, NORTHERN IRELAND

www.ambassador-international.com

SAVE YOURSELF SOME THERAPY
Four Dangers to Our Mental Health and What to Do About It

Hardcover ISBN: 978-1-64960-705-8
Paperback ISBN: 978-1-64960-706-5
eISBN: 978-1-64960-719-5

Cover design by Karen Slayne
Interior Typesetting by Dentelle Design
Editing by Sara Johnson
Author photo credit Jessica Barley

Ambassador International titles may be purchased in bulk for education, business, fundraising, or sales promotional use. For information, please email sales@emeraldhouse.com.

AMBASSADOR INTERNATIONAL
Emerald House
411 University Ridge, Suite B14
Greenville, SC 29601
United States
www.ambassador-international.com

AMBASSADOR BOOKS
The Mount
2 Woodstock Link
Belfast, BT6 8DD
Northern Ireland, United Kingdom
www.ambassadormedia.co.uk

The colophon is a trademark of Ambassador, a Christian publishing company.

For Greg, who helped me brainstorm all the concepts

in this book evening upon evening—we did it

For my sons, you make me stronger, better—thank you

Table of Contents

Foreword

Last month, my wife and I were sitting on a plane waiting for takeoff when the pilot announced there would be a delay. The mechanics were doing some preventative maintenance, so the plane was not prepared to fly. My wife and I were not excited about the interruption to our flight plans! We were within hours of finishing a series of flights that had taken us literally around the world. We were tired and eager to get home to sleep in our own bed.

But we were also eager to get home—alive! So, whatever time the mechanical team needed to increase the chance of a safe flight, we fully supported it. Preventative care can seem unnecessary or even frustrating when it requires rescheduling our plans or reevaluating our priorities. But the alternative is even more unpleasant. This seems obvious when we compare safe flights with plane crashes, but perhaps this is not as obvious in the mundane rhythms of life.

Amber Bateman is like a wise pilot who encourages us to unbuckle our seatbelt for a time, relax, and do some lifestyle "maintenance." This pause may seem unnecessary, but it could result in some new ways of thinking and living that lead to lifelong flourishing.

Amber invites us to slow down, declutter, compete less, and value community. She refuses to leave these enhancements in the realm of the theoretical but includes lots of practical action steps in each chapter such as helpful book recommendations, practicing Sabbath, spending time outdoors, and "souplication"—a soul-nourishing practice she and some friends invented during graduate school.

Best of all, Amber repeatedly points us to Jesus, Who cares so deeply about the health of our souls, not just the deadlines we think we must meet. God provides the grace we need, and His Word supplies the guidance we crave.

So sit back and relax. Let's do some much-needed preventative care. The trip will be so much more enjoyable when we apply these safety measures!

—**Peter Hubbard**

Teaching Pastor at North Hills Church, Taylors, South Carolina

and Author of *Love Into Light*

CHAPTER 0

The Problem

(It is really an introduction; but I want you to actually read it, so I'm calling it Chapter 0 in hopes that maybe you will.)

"In today's culture, what we consider to be normal . . . in fact undermines health and promotes disease. So that illness itself, whether of mind or body, is in many cases a normal response to abnormal circumstances."[1]
—Gabor Maté

As a mental health counselor, I get the privilege of sitting with people in difficult seasons, who face challenging situations that don't always have answers. I love what I do. I find people fascinating—how we get into trouble; how we respond to trouble; and of course, how we recover from trouble. And trouble we have.

In many ways, we are more blessed and fortunate in modern Western society than ever before. We have access to state-of-the-art health care, and we can travel literally across the world in twenty-four

---

1   "Gabor Maté: "Healing into Wholeness in a Toxic Culture," Sounds True(podcast), December 20, 2022, https://resources.soundstrue.com/podcast/gabor-mate-a-personal-view-of-healing-into-wholeness-in-a-toxic-culture.

hours. Through a mysterious, invisible form of communication called the internet, we have access to an amount of information never before imagined. We can learn a new skill or find an answer to most any question in the span of seconds—from a device that we take with us wherever we go. With this development has come incredible opportunities and resources previously unimagined; stuff that would leave our great, great grandparents in awe.

But do all of these advances come without any risk? I would argue that we live in a time in history that is extremely dangerous to our mental health. We are in trouble. Mental health problems continue to rise. Chronic stress, anxiety, depression, substance use disorders, sexual addictions, relationship conflict, attention difficulties, and other mental illnesses abound. It is rare to meet someone who doesn't know a family member, friend, or coworker who is struggling in one of these areas. According to Mental Health America, in 2023, it is estimated that 17 percent to 29 percent of adult Americans struggle with a mental health illness (not including substance use).Fifteen percent of Americans report having a substance use disorder, and 4 percent report serious thoughts of suicide.[2]

What is causing such a drastic increase in mental health problems? Is it simply, as some would suggest, that we are just talking about it more? Is it that we are more loosely defining "mental health problems"? Are we just more sensitive or too privileged to have "real" problems? Possibly. The answers to these questions are, of course, complex and multi-dimensional. There are countless factors that affect why one person struggles the way they do, while another person in a

---

2   "Adult Data 2023," Mental Health America, last modified 2024, https://www. mhanational.org/the-state-of-mental-health-in-america/archived-reports.

similar situation seems to fair just fine. There are physical factors such as genetics, brain chemistry, environmental toxins, and head injuries. There are social elements such as family of origin dynamics, parenting styles, economic status, and cultural nuances. Traumatic events, personal choice, spiritual warfare, and an unknown number of additional factors can all play a role in the way humans struggle with their thoughts, feelings, and behaviors (the components that make up mental health).

I believe there are some significant cultural factors—four in particular—that are silent killers to mental health in modern America. These modern dangers will likely be no surprise to anyone. They are things we know are probably not good for us, but we do not take them that seriously. We believe we have more important things to worry about, so we do not give these aspects of our culture much attention. Or we may know they are dangerous but do not believe there is anything we can do about it. Perhaps some will think, "That's just life."

Each danger on its own does not necessarily have to be reason for great concern. They are harmless enough in small doses. The problem is that, for many people, the doses are not small. These cultural dangers are woven into the fabric of many people's way of life; and without realizing it, we can find ourselves swept away with mental health problems and feeling at a loss as to where they came from or how they became so serious. Then, if we consider all four of these dangers combined, we are talking about a very dangerous (some have suggested toxic) environment for our minds.

We know that there is some benefit to eating healthy, exercising, and getting good sleep for our physical health. We accept that germs exist and that if you lick doorknobs in public buildings, you increase your chances of catching an illness (and also being stared at). What if there are things we do—ideas we believe—that tear down our mental immune system? If we are not aware of the dangers, it is hard to stay on the offensive; and we find ourselves in a professional's office again.

The title of this book may cause one to wonder if the author is against therapy, complaining about it, or suggesting it is not helpful. That is not the case. I love being a professional counselor because I believe in this work. I see people getting better; managing their symptoms in a healthy way; and finding freedom, meaning, and restored relationships as they do hard work in therapy. Professional therapy is a gift, and most people could benefit from it at some point in their lives. There should be absolutely no shame in getting help.

But therapy is not the only solution, nor must it be a long-term one. Professional help is likely to be a very wise option for nearly all of us at some point in our lives, but I believe there are preventative measures— lifestyle changes that can be applied up front to help mitigate damage to our mental health. Even if you applied all the principles in this book, professional counseling may still be a good idea for you; and the two can certainly work hand in hand.

I like to compare mental health to dental health for a better understanding. Many factors can influence the health of one's teeth. Some factors are not in one's control—genetics for example. And some we can have more control over—whether or not to eat candy every night before falling asleep. No matter the cause, sometimes you need help from a professional to care for your teeth in a way you are not qualified or willing to perform on yourself. However, there are things you can do—practices you can adopt—to maintain good dental hygiene and reduce your risks of more serious complications. That is what I attempt to address in this book concerning mental health—hygiene practices that require work and intentionality but that I trust you will find well worth the effort.

This little book outlines four dangers which our modern culture poses to our mental health and some practical ideas about what to do differently. Please, do not get overwhelmed by the "what to do about it" sections. Entire books have been written about these topics, so see them as challenges to explore, not as things you must master all at once. As I write this book, I am mostly picturing my female American clients and friends; however, I hope that anyone living in modern cultures around the world can relate to and be inspired by this book. As a counselor, it is my passion to help people walk through life's difficulties with hope and practical help. This work is not meant to be an exhaustive study. This is a brief guide with two main goals:

- To provide a platform for dialoging about mental health (a topic which affects so many, and yet many are not talking about it with real people in their daily lives).
- To inspire change as readers reflect, read more resources, and act.

Please consider reading the suggested resources at the end of each chapter. They are excellent reads that have been monumental in my ongoing journey toward mental health. The book is designed to be worked through as an individual or in a small group (a workplace team or church small group, for example). The accompanying discussion questions are intentional and encourage deep, meaningful discussion. This edition you are reading is written for Christians in particular.

Although I do not know you personally or all the factors that influence your mental health, I am hopeful and confident that if you apply the principles in this book, you really could "save yourself some therapy." Again, that is not to say you should not go to therapy (some of you may decide that is exactly what you should do after reading this book), but rather that if and when you go, you will already be ahead. You will have eliminated, or at least become aware of, the cultural dangers that may be exasperating your personal struggles. You will be equipped to make better use of your time with a therapist.

Jesus came that we "may have life and have it abundantly,"³ and that is my sincere hope for this project—that it may bring us closer to Jesus and each other as we seek abundant life together.

---

3   John 10:10

CHAPTER 1
Danger One: Hurriedness

"Hurry is the great enemy of spiritual life in our day.
You must ruthlessly eliminate hurry from your life."[4]

—Dallas Willard

W e live in a fast culture. Speed matters. It matters a lot. Do it quicker; do it more efficiently; this is the cry of nearly every aspect of modern life: from business, transportation, and education; to food, spirituality, and family life. Even modern "leisure" can be in a hurry. But it has not always been this way.

In his book, *In Praise of Slowness*, journalist Carl Honore explores the history of how modern Western society came to be so obsessed with speed. He highlights cultural changes brought upon by industrial and technological revolutions. He walks readers through how inventions such as the mechanical clock in the 1400s and the steam engine in the 1700s made way for a global standard time and established punctuality as a moral virtue near the beginning of the 1900s.[5] Honore makes a case

---

4   Dallas Willard quoted by John Mark Comer, *The Ruthless Elimination of Hurry* (Colorado Springs: WaterBrook, 2019).
5   Carl Honore, *In Praise of Slowness: Challenging the Cult of Speed* (New York: HarperOne, 2005).

for why faster is not always better, and we can absolutely see this as true when it comes to mental health in modern life.

Many Americans are experiencing high levels of anxiety, and those levels are not going down. The pressures and stresses of life—they continue to press. For many families, life just seems to get faster and faster. I have met with many people who have all the makings of a "good life"—spouse and kids, job, house, favorite restaurant within walking distance, two dogs, and a seasonal pass to college football games. They plop down into my office utterly exhausted and exhale. They have not slept well, have not had a meaningful conversation with their spouse in days, snapped at their kids too many times, and stress-ate more pints of ice cream than they care to admit. And they cannot keep their minds from spinning with a thousand things they need to do once the fifty minutes of therapy is up.

In some ways, the 2020 COVID-19 pandemic slowed many families down; and social media posts emerged with cries to "remember what we've learned." There were pleas to not jump right back into the crazy cycle, to take time with the family and friends that matter the most to us, to make meals at home and stop racing around to twenty different activities in one day. Yet post-pandemic life has led to new problems for some. For example, the rise of remote workers has only brought a temptation to eat lunch in front of our laptops, to take a quick online class or shoot out a few emails while we scarf down a microwaved lunch even in our own home. Many have found themselves right back to a place of hustle and bustle that leaves them exhausted. It continues to take a toll. "I just can't keep up with it all," clients tell me.

I have been there, too. As a conscientious, task-oriented, perfectionist-prone, achiever personality, I have been the worst at this!

Hurry is my natural banner cry. I can really get things done! Getting stuff done fuels me and will likely always be a part of my natural tendency. However, becoming a counselor and balancing a professional career with family and inner personal life has caused me to question, "Why do I really need to rush, anyway?"

There is so much to do, we say. We must get things done. We must earn money. We must earn *more* money. Time is money. And we treat it as such. We talk about spending time, wasting time, saving time, buying time, and even killing time. As a culture, we all feel this invisible hand behind us—sometimes shoving, sometimes a soft nudge, but always pressure. Pressure to get ahead. Pressure to catch up on something. We constantly feel a need to get ahead while also feeling chronically behind.

Even when we know we should slow down or want to slow down, we cannot. We do not know how. Many of us are addicted to speed. We are so accustomed to fast food, fast shipping, fast internet, and fast bedtime stories with our kids. We believe we must drive fast, work fast, and get better—fast. Going slow can feel so unnatural, sacrilegious even, to our cultural value of hurry. Most of us do not want to go back to ancient times before we had these very convenient resources, but we also realize that we desperately need strategies to maintain a healthy balance.

The hurriedness of our culture leaves many of us feeling continuously behind in life and feeling the need to "get our life together." And we are killing ourselves in the process. Our mental, physical, and relational health constantly takes a hit. We have so much knowledge about how to get healthy and stay healthy. In a lot of ways, we know what we need to do. But as I sit with clients discussing what could save their marriages, decrease their anxieties, and help relieve depression, the problem is often the same—*I don't have enough time*—or money, but often it is time. "I know I should exercise, but when? I am barely keeping up as it is. If you add one more thing to my to do list, I am going to really lose it."

Living this way can have obvious effects on our mental health. Chronic hurriedness leads to chronic stress, which keeps us in fight or flight mode with our heart rate elevated, mind racing, and cortisol hormones flooding our body. The sympathetic nervous system that is designed to benefit us in a crisis becomes a way of life. Being in a rush makes us more physically tense and more irritable with our loved ones, especially children.

Children, by the way, are naturally slow. They want to be held, to touch your face, to stick their dirty fingers up your nose for no productive reason at all, and giggle about it endlessly. Parents know that during the walk from the car to the doctor's appointment (that you are probably late to), children stop to examine a shiny, bent paperclip or the remains of an unlucky squirrel skeleton. We pull at their arms and say, "Uh huh. That's nice, honey. But come on; we must go." And we keep going. And going. Because when the doctor's visit is over, that child knows that their loving parent will haul them along to the next thing until they collapse in bed, get up, and do it all over again.

I have heard parents say that we need to teach children how to "make it" in the world; if you want to be successful, you have to hustle— now. I have said it myself. But we must ask ourselves: do we really want to teach our kids to hustle all the time? That faster is better and being slow is a sin? Do we want to teach our children this unhealthy cultural way of life?

A note about children: any of the dangers we are addressing here apply to children as well, and even more so. Children are especially vulnerable to unhealthy practices. While there is a very popular belief that "children are resilient," it is not really true. Children are *adaptable*. They do not bounce back to their original state (as the term resilience means); but rather, they mold and adapt their brains with new information and experiences. "Normal" unhealthy habits for children do not make them stronger; it just makes unhealthy habits normal. We have a responsibility and opportunity to protect and prepare our kids to make healthy choices for their mental and emotional health.

So what is the alternative to a culture of hurriedness? *Slowing down and being present.* By slowing down, I do not mean we all quit our jobs and move to a deserted island. By slowing down, I do not necessarily mean that you should never have a busy day. Busy days, where life circumstances require a lot of your time and attention, will happen to all of us. Cars break down; children wake up with a fever; ankles get sprained; milk gets spilled; stuff happens that we cannot always control. And those things can make our day busy—full of needs that need to be met.

Busy is not the same as *hurried*. Busy is what we just described in the paragraph above. We have responsibilities that should be tended to. By this definition, busyness has always existed since the dawn of time. Bodies need to be cleaned; people need to be fed;and homes need to be built. That is not the same thing as modern hurriedness. By hurriedness, I mean what we have referred to in previous paragraphs in this chapter: that uneasy, antsy feeling that you are behind and that you and everyone around you needs to move faster. Being unnecessarily busy can, of course, lead to being hurried, and the strategies ahead will address that; but there is an important distinction to make because I am arguing that one can be busy (have a lot of responsibilities) without being constantly hurried. The difference is being present—mindful of where you actually are in the moment—rather than living in the future.

Stress is the pressure we feel in the moment to rise to a challenge or perform a certain way. All of us will face stressful situations in our lives. That is part of life, and we have responsibilities we must tend to. But in light of the danger of a fast culture, we have to ask ourselves these questions: Is all of the stress I'm experiencing necessary? Is any of it an amount God is *not* calling me to? Can any of it be reduced without compromising what God *is* calling me to do?

Anxiety is the negative thoughts, feelings, and bodily sensations we experience even when we are not in immediate danger at that moment. Usually, we are experiencing anxiety about something that is in the past or future, not in that present moment. We can reduce a significant amount of anxiety by being present and coming back to right here and right now.

Let us look at an example to further illustrate this concept.

Hurried

You have an appointment to meet with a friend at a coffee shop in fifteen minutes. You leave work in a fluster, even though the coffee shop is only ten minutes away. As you drive toward the coffee shop, you look at your phone at stop lights to catch up on emails and look at cat memes. You arrive at the coffee shop and notice there are no seats left, so you quickly text your friend that there are no seats and ask if she wants to go somewhere else.

Your friend arrives and says we do not have time to go anywhere else, and you begin talking about how busy you both are. You get to the counter and feel flustered because you do not know what you want, and you are irritated that the line was so long, anyway. You make some small talk with your friend; but really, all you can think about is how much work you must do when you get back to the office.

PRESENT

You have an appointment to meet with a friend at a coffee shop in fifteen minutes. You take a minute to pause whatever work you are doing and jot down on a sticky note where you need to resume when you return. You look around your office, take a deep breath, and walk out to your car. You take the ten-minute drive to the coffee shop to check in with yourself. *How am I feeling? What would I like to discuss with my friend when I see her?*

You notice it is a beautiful winter day: cold and crisp but sunny. You arrive at the coffee shop and notice there are no seats left; but it does not bother you because it's a beautiful day, and standing in the sunshine outside might actually be nice. Your friend arrives, and you greet each other with a hug and genuine, "How are you?" You both ask meaningful questions to each other as you wait in line. You order your drinks and enjoy them so much that you decide a London Fog is your new favorite drink. You leave the coffee date feeling encouraged and energized for the rest of your workday.

Which of these two examples do you relate to more often? When was the last time you were fully present in the moment—where you felt fully alive and fully engaged in real time with real people without any kind of cyber world or thinking into the future? This difference is significant and is a great contributor to overall mental health.

BIBLICAL PERSPECTIVE

In his book, *The Ruthless Elimination of Hurry,* John Mark Comer challenges readers with this question: "Was Jesus ever in a hurry?"[6] He certainly had busy days, days where there were lots of things to be done: people to heal, life-changing messages to preach, humankind to save for eternity—small things like that. Surely, He was busy at times, but was He *hurried?* Was He put out—emotionally deregulated—His mind off thinking about how it was nearly sundown, and He needed to get here and there?

It is hard to think of a passage in Scripture that we find Jesus in a rush. Was it because He did not have anything pressing to do? Of course not. We look at the Gospels and find that when Jesus' friend was deathly ill, He stayed two days longer. He did not rush off.[7] Another time, we see Jesus on His way to heal a very sick girl, and what does He do? He stops to ask who touched Him in the crowd.[8]

---

6   John Mark Comer, *The Ruthless Elimination of Hurry* (Colorado Springs: WaterBrook, 2019).
7   John 11:1-45
8   Mark 5:25-34

I am not arguing that it is wrong to rush to your friend's bedside if he is ill but just pointing out that Jesus was intentional, present, and focused, even in the face of immediate suffering and need. When the Lord walked this earth, He displayed to us a way of being present, being aware of, and being concerned about the task His Father was asking of Him right there in that present moment.

Yes, He knew the future was coming; and yes, He was planning and thinking about eternity past and eternity future. But He lived in the time and space (which He created) to be fully available to the people in that space. These observations beg the question: if Jesus (when here in physical humanity) was not routinely rushed and hurried, why are we? Do we have more important things to do than Jesus?

The Ruthless Elimination of Hurry also addresses the fact that Jesus did not try to "do it all."[9] He did not write a book; He did not command a military army; and He did not own a vehicle or house. Yet He was the most successful, most perfect human to ever walk the earth. He was the most productive in fulfilling the purpose for which He came. Why do so many of us believe that if we do not do "all the things" that we have failed? We will continue to explore this question as we work through this book. For now, let us address some common objections to slowing down.

OBJECTION 1: I LIKE BEING BUSY

"What if I like being busy?" some of you may ask. "What if I *need* to be busy?" What about those who need to be busy to help stay out of trouble or curb loneliness? Is staying busy doing positive things not better than sitting at home feeling sorry for myself or doing things I should not? I

---

9   John Mark Comer, *The Ruthless Elimination of Hurry* (Colorado Springs: WaterBrook, 2019).

hear you. Yes, I do think that some people may find that staying active and having a full schedule is actually beneficial for their mental health. Some people, especially those struggling with depression, may need to find more meaningful things to do. But again, having a full life is not the same as *hurriedness*. The antidote to hurriedness is not boredom or laziness; it is being present where you are and who are with at that given time. Anyone can benefit from this.

OBJECTION 2: ESCAPE

Many find they keep themselves going from one thing to the next without pause because when they do slow down, they find themselves flooded with anxiety, negative thoughts, and overwhelming feelings. We can use hurriedness to avoid having to face our external and internal problems.

"This is how I survive," you may say. "It works, doesn't it?" Yes. And no. Yes, because sometimes a season of life is just plain hard, and we need to keep moving—keep doing the next right thing. But even in those times, I would still not recommend hurriedness and frantically going through your days disoriented and out of touch with yourself and others.

If you have a physical sickness such as a runny nose, cough, or fever, distracting yourself with a movie or some music can be okay and even a healthy way to cope. But if after six months, you are still watching TV and ignoring the fact that you have had a fever for months, something is wrong. At that point, masking your symptoms with distractions is not wise. It is time to address what is going on with you. It is time to consider getting help—going to a professional doctor or talking with trusted family and friends.

Unfortunately, many people live this way in regard to their mental health. They have chronic mental health symptoms that are begging to be addressed; but instead, they continue to distract themselves, staying so busy that they do not have time to think about the fact that they have had a "fever" for six months. Friend, if this is you, please, please slow down and get help. Your problem is not likely to resolve itself. I know it can seem overwhelming, but you can do this. Let us get into some more practical ways to protect ourselves against the modern danger of hurriedness.

LEARN THE ART OF SAYING NO

A large part of slowing down is going to include reducing your schedule and number of obligations. Saying no is an important first step. "No, thank you, I can't come to that party." "No, unfortunately I will not be able to volunteer with that fundraiser this year." "No, even though that job would make me more money, the extended nights and weekend hours are not worth my mental health and the health of my family."

You do not have to say yes to every request that is asked of you or to every opportunity that comes your way. Simplifying your schedule and responsibilities will greatly help make space for breathing room in your life. This is a simple concept but quite hard for many people to do.

LEARN TO SET HEALTHY BOUNDARIES

Own the fact that managing your time is your responsibility. We are accountable to how we spend our God-given resources. Stop blaming your hurriedness on your job, your kids, your in-laws, your finances, and so on. Accept that we live in a fast culture that will pull our time and attention in one hundred different ways every single day if we let it. We can complain all we want (and our complaints are valid), but nothing will change until we take ownership over our own pace of life. See the recommended resource section for some books about healthy boundaries.

KNOW YOUR PRIORITIES

Once I was complaining to a friend about how busy I was and that I did not have time to do something healthy for me.

She told me, "Amber, you will always have time for the things that are most important to you."

I thought, *No, you do not understand. I really do not have enough time.*

But she was right. I might not have time to do everything that I *want* to do or *feel* is important, but I have to practice triage with my time. In a culture where we have a thousand choices and endless opportunities, saying no to one thing is a yes to something else. Do you long for more time with your family? Saying no to checking your Instagram feed can mean a yes to shooting some hoops with your son, even if it is only for a few minutes.

ADDRESS PERFECTIONISM IN YOUR LIFE AND LEARN TO ACCEPT YOUR FINITENESS

Jesus did not do it all while He was here on this earth, and neither can you. Accept the fact that you are not a superhero, and that is okay. In *The Ruthless Elimination of Hurry*, Comer challenges us to consider that Jesus chose to take on a human form that was finite.[10] He got tired.

---

10   John Mark Comer, *The Ruthless Elimination of Hurry* (Colorado Springs: Water-Brook, 2019).

He got hungry. He sweat and cried and felt abandoned.[11] There is a lot of freedom to be found in accepting that we are not gods.

PRACTICE SABBATH

Rest is something many modern people really struggle to do. We like being in control or, at least, the illusion of being in control. We are really good at being entertained and amused but not necessarily resting. This is not just a holy command, but it is also a really good idea. Consider starting your journey to a less hurried life by slowing down at least one day a week. Not all slow days need to be a Sabbath, but all Sabbaths should be slow days.

TAKE NAPS

Jesus did. Or at least lie down somewhere without music playing or the TV going and just close your eyes. If you want, experiment with lying on your stomach or on your back with a blanket or pillow on your chest. Tune into the sounds and sensations you feel right there in that moment. Practice some deep breathing if you feel anxious or restless.

ASK GOD REGULARLY HOW HE WANTS YOU TO SPEND YOUR ALLOTTED TIME ON EARTH

There are countless things you could do in any given day. Many of them are very good endeavors: feed the hungry, shelter the homeless, bring the gospel to an unreached people group, foster and adopt children, or master a craft in music or art. Maybe I am naïve as to what

---

11   Matthew 8:24; Matthew 4:2; Luke 22:44; John 11:35; Mark 15:34

kind of superpower you hold; but very likely, God is not calling you to do all those things today—or maybe not even in your lifetime. Slow down and become laser-focused on what God has for you each day. As Annie Dillard said, "For of course, how we spend our days is how we spend our lives."[12]

STOP TRYING TO FILL EVERY MOMENT WITH SOMETHING "PRODUCTIVE" OR EXCITING

Some of you will not struggle with this; but to those who do, stop driving all around town, going from store to store, trying to accomplish too many things in one afternoon. Not too long ago, my husband and I were on a date. We picked a restaurant we wanted to go to and looked up when they opened. Upon realizing we had thirteen minutes to kill before the restaurant opened, our immediate response was, "Are there any stores close by? Is there anything we need to buy while we have time?"

It was a defining moment for us. We looked at each other and realized we did not have to rush around and try to fill thirteen minutes. What if we—gasp!—got to the restaurant thirteen minutes early and just sat in the car, talking and observing life around us? Would that really be so bad? (Spoiler alert: it was not.)

PRACTICE BEING CONTENT AND LET FOMO (FEAR OF MISSING OUT) GO

We cannot have it all or do it all without a cost. When people hear that I have two small children and that we are a two-working-parent household, they assume, "You must be so busy!" But truthfully, my

---

12   Annie Dillard, *The Writing Life* (New York: Harper Perennial, 2013).

husband and I have worked hard not to be very busy. We are currently saying no to several good activities that would make our lives too hurried. We do not go to the gym; we do not have any pets; we do not watch TV more than a couple times a month; we do not play video games; we do not currently have hobbies outside of things we can do at home once the kids are asleep; we do not play sports or go to sporting events. Of course, I am not saying there is anything wrong with those things or that we never have done them. The point is that we've said no to a lot of things right now so we can say yes to the things that are most important to us, such as quality time with our kids and for us as a couple every day. There is great freedom in finding contentment in the season you are currently in without trying to do everything.

RELEASE YOURSELF FROM THE PRESSURE TO LIVE "BIG"

Author and blogger Mandy McCarty Harris had two daughters who died of neurogenerative diseases when they were seven and eleven years old. She would know something about wanting to make the most of the time she had. She encourages others to let go of the pressure to make every day memorable and to "live like you were dying." She says, "Lay down the urgency to make every day the best day ever. The treasures of life are found in ordinary moments, with the people you love, and you don't have to rush that."[13]

SIMPLIFY YOUR POSSESSIONS

We live in a very consumeristic culture. So much time and mental energy goes into accumulating more stuff. Consider the amount

---

13   Leslie Means, *So God Made a Mother* (Carol Stream, Illinois: Tyndale, 2023), 18.

of time we spend thinking about the things we want to buy and researching the best kind of that thing. Then we look at advertisements, browse sales, and purchase the item (and possibly return the item). But we are not done: we must clean and maintain the item, buy more items to go with our new item, and take on extra hours at work to pay for our new item! Modern shopping can be a colossal waste of time that continually pulls our resources away from what we really value. When you have a free moment, resist the urge to browse online shopping sites or stop by a store. Living a more minimalist lifestyle can provide a lot of extra space in your schedule, in your budget, and in your garage.

BECOME MORE HOME (AND LOCAL NEIGHBORHOOD) CENTERED

I have heard this tip from a few social medias low-living bloggers, and I have found it to be true. So many modern Americans do not spend a lot of time in their homes and neighborhoods. In fact, many spend a lot of time in the car, going to work, school, extracurricular activities, restaurants, concerts, shopping centers, and pretty much anywhere but home. If you really want to slow down your pace of life and decrease your stress, try spending more time at home. This does not mean you have to be isolated or antisocial; invite family, friends, and neighbors over for a meal or to play a board game. Regularly take walks around your neighborhood and wave to your neighbors. Start a small garden in your front yard so you can be available to chat with neighbors if they walk by. Be intentional about simplifying your possessions and making your home a rejuvenating place to be, rather than just a place to hold all your junk. It does not need to take a lot of money or skill to improve the atmosphere of your home. Start by decluttering stuff you do not need and set up thoughtful spaces that promote relaxation and quality time with others.

WALK OR BIKE INSTEAD OF DRIVE, IF YOU CAN

In his book, *The Little Book of Lykke,* Meik Wiking notes that happy people (people who report being more satisfied with their lives) often choose walking or riding their bikes as their preferred mode of transportation. "Part of the reason we feel in a better mood when cycling rather than driving is that our senses are more engaged. We simply feel more alive—walking is a more sensual experience than driving."[14]

By "sensual," Wiking is referring to being more in tune with the senses. If walking or biking for your daily activities is just not doable for you, consider driving a slower route with the windows rolled down. This can give you similar benefits to walking or biking because it is more grounding, meaning that you are engaging your five senses (sight, smell, hearing, taste, and touch), which can help you be more present in the moment and reduce mental clutter and anxiety.

STOP AT RED LIGHTS WHEN DRIVING

Do not just stop your car; stop your "productivity" as well. Resist the urge to check your phone. Use the opportunity to take a deep breath, check in with yourself, gather your thoughts, or talk to the Lord. Commutes are a wonderful opportunity to allow your soul (your thoughts and emotions) to catch up with your physical body.

---

14   Meik Wiking, *The Little Book of Lykke: Secrets of the World's Happiest People* (New York: Harper Collins, 2017), 147.

Most red lights in the United States are designed to last sixty to ninety seconds—less than a minute and a half.[15] Trying to cram in random "productivity" into that time is not worth the risk to your safety or your mental space.

Reduce Time-consuming Media and Especially Media on the Internet

Spend more time being present with the people who are physically with you (much more on this in the next chapter). If you are looking for something to watch, try getting a movie from the local library instead of scrolling through dozens of options on a streaming service. Or trade an hour of overstimulating, low-quality media with a wholesome twenty-minute show you are actually interested in on YouTube, for example.

Practice Mindfulness, Meditation, and Grounding Exercises

There are many resources on this topic and some from a Christian perspective. This could be a whole book in itself, but you can begin by simply looking up deep breathing or grounding exercises online.

Spend Time in Nature

Become more aware of and attuned to the seasons. Is it summer? Take advantage of fireflies, sitting by the lake, and fresh fruit. Is it

---

15   "Signal Cycle Lengths," National Association of City Transportation Officials, Accessed June 28, 2025, https://nacto.org/publication/urban-street-design-guide/intersection-design-elements/traffic-signals/signal-cycle-lengths.

winter? Cozy up with some good books or indoor projects. Take a five-minute break in the afternoon to go out in a parking lot at your work and soak in a few minutes of sunlight. More on why time in nature is therapeutic in a future chapter.

ENGAGE IN SLOW ACTIVITIES

Baking, playing an instrument, or singing or whistling are excellent examples of slow activities. Do something outside, such as take a walk, garden, or fish. These are ancient practices that humans have been engaging in for thousands of years and call us back to a more humane existence. Find a hobby that requires you to sit still and create something with your hands. Some ideas include knitting, blacksmithing, origami, carving wood, sketching, pottery, leatherwork, soap making, jewelry making, and painting. Try reading physical books and particularly children's books with illustrations.

ENGAGE IN MONO TASKING

This is simply the opposite of that great American pastime—multitasking. Instead of trying to kill two birds with one stone and get as many things as possible done at once, experiment with just focusing on one task at a time. If you are on a lunch break at work, try simply eating your meal and observing your surroundings. Resist the temptation to look up something, scroll social media, pay a bill online, or respond to non-emergency texts. You may be fascinated, as I was, that the whole world did not implode into a million pieces because I slowed down long enough to dedicate fifteen uninterrupted minutes of my life to simply eating my lunch. In fact, you may discover that you become more productive, more alive, and more useful to others.

I had been mulling over the title of this book for months. I knew the subtitle pretty early on, but that main title was out of my reach long after I began writing the book. One lunch break at work, I started to pull up a YouTube video on my computer as I sat down with my microwaved leftovers. It occurred to me that there really was not anything I wanted to watch and that instead I should simply eat my lunch. I opened the window of my office to let in some fresh air and munched away as I gazed at the weeds in the empty lot behind our office. To my surprise and amusement, a groundhog poked his head out of the weeds and stared at me. I smiled, and it immediately came to me. *Save yourself some therapy.*

"That's it," I muttered to myself.

I am convinced that the Lord gave me the title to this book right at the moment that I actually applied what I was inviting others to do. I slowed down, and the inspiration came.

REFLECTIVE QUESTIONS:

1. Do you think hurriedness is a problem for our culture?
2. In what ways/areas of your life do you struggle with hurriedness?
3. Are there any areas of your life where you feel you are pretty good at being present? What helps you be able to be more present in those times?
4. Do you know anyone who is particularly strong in the area of being present and not being hurried?

5. What hesitations or objections do you have to slowing down and being more present?

6. What is one small (or large) step you could take to practice slowing down and being more present?

RECOMMENDED RESOURCES:

- *The Ruthless Elimination of Hurry* by John Mark Comer (Christian perspective)

- *In the Praise of Slowness* by Carl Honore

CHAPTER 2

Danger Two: Overstimulation

"There is a simple free way to improve mental health: put down the phone and do something else."[16]

—Jean Twenge

It is 4:00 p.m. Time for me to go home. *I gotta get home. Make dinner. Spend time with my husband and kids.* I mutter to myself as I look around my counseling office turning off lights and grabbing my things. *Don't forget your laptop charger in the wall . . . Don't forget the charger . . .*

But wow, my head hurts. And it takes me some intentional self-reflection to even identify what I feel—physically and emotionally. Really, it just feels like . . . ugh. Blah. I am cranky. Irritable. *What's wrong? Nothing. Nothing is wrong. I did a good job today. No one is suicidal. My notes are done. So why do I feel so—what's the word—frazzled?*

A dozen thoughts swirl in my head as I continue to close up: *What do I have to do when I get home? I need to respond to that family text conversation.*

---

16   Jean Twenge, *iGen. Why Today's Super Connected Kids Are Growing Up Less Rebellious, More Tolerant, Less Happy, and Completely Unprepared for Adulthood* (New York: Atria Books, 2018).

I forgot to send that email. What will I wear to that upcoming event? Oh, yeah, I did see a cute dress on social media—I wonder how long it's on sale.

I switch the sign on my door indicating I am done for the day. But am I?

Six hours later, I am sitting up in my bed, looking at that dress on my phone. But by now, three more ads for similar dresses have caught my eye. *Ahh, I like the color on this one, but this one is cheaper and available in a local store so I can try it on first.* My head still hurts.

No doubt, being a professional counselor is a mentally and emotionally taxing job; but we are not the only ones whose brains feel fuzzy on an average day. Hurriedness is a problem and overstimulation its sidekick.

THE PROBLEM

I was a communications major in undergraduate school. In journalism class, we learned that the more stimulating the story—the more sensations, emotions, and mental images you can evoke—the more attention the article is likely to receive; and it is more likely to be remembered. The more the attention, the more views, the more likes, the more shares, the more "successful" the article.

It has been claimed that Americans are exposed to several thousand advertisements per day. Some have questioned that number as ridiculously extreme and not backed up by any actual research. One informal experiment counted ninety-three ads per day,[17] and I think this more accurately describes average exposure. But obviously, the

---

17   Sam Anderson, "How Many Ads do We Really See in a Day: Spoiler, It's Not 10,000," *The Drum*, May 3, 2023,https://www.thedrum.com/news/2023/05/03/how-many-ads-do-we-really-see-day-spoiler-it-s-not-10000.

truth varies widely depending on where you live, work, and play—the routines of your daily life. But whatever the accurate statistic, it cannot be denied that we are bombarded with a lot of advertisements and a lot of stimulation in general.

Our modern economy thrives on stimulation. Most commercial media outlets are specifically designed to produce as much dopamine as possible in consumers. Dopamine is a neurotransmitter (sending messages from the brain throughout other parts of the body) and the "pleasure hormone" (associated with eating sugar, being sexually aroused, winning a game, or experiencing a drug high). Many large companies now have positions for behavioral scientists whose job is to research human and social behavior. This provides companies with valuable information that can be used to benefit the company. More knowledge about what humans want and how they think and feel is more knowledge about how to keep employees or how to better market products to potential consumers.

Successful modern marketing strategies are researched and designed to be *addictive* in order to keep us coming back for more. Have you ever been thinking about buying something (say a puppy, for example), only to discover the very next day that your entire social media feed is peppered with the most beautiful photos of the most adorable Golden Retriever pups you have ever seen? Creepy, right? But what is even creepier to me is that so many times, it works. I find myself thinking about that thing and feeling grumpy if I can't get it as soon as possible.

Our attention is constantly being pulled so many different ways in a given day. Consider the fact that most of us have minicomputers with an unlimited amount of information in our pockets. *In. Our. Pockets.*

Access is available at any given point throughout the day. Reports vary, but many claim that the average American adult (in 2023) looks at their phone 144 times per day and spends over four hours a day on their devices.[18] Some studies show that the iGen generation (those born between 1995 and 2012) spend more than that—at least six hours a day on their phones.[19] I am always leery of the accuracy of statistics, but the point here is clear—we spend a lot of time on our phones.

We see it all the time, right? We are in the checkout line at the grocery store, the waiting room at the doctor's office, before the church service starts, and even in my therapy office. Some clients' phones are constantly binging; and they are pulled, as if by force, to gaze over at their devices. Many pick up their phones, apologize, and then proceed to respond to whatever cannot wait fifty minutes for them to finish their session. I have been there, too.

It is not just that our phones are binging frequently. I find myself checking my phone even when it is not making noise. Just whenever I have a spare moment, I can be caught cradling it in my hand and gazing at it like Gollum with the ring of power from *The Lord of the Rings*. Am I the only one who thinks this is incredibly messed up? I, for one, do not like the idea of treating an electronic device like I am in a relationship with it. Catherine Price said it well in her "Open Letter to My Phone":

> Phone, you amaze me. I mean that literally: not only do you allow me to travel across time and space, but I'm amazed by how many nights I've stayed up three hours past my bedtime

---

18   Alex Kerai, "Cell Phone Use Statistics: Mornings Are for Notifications," *Reviews. org*, July 21, 2023, https://www.reviews.org/mobile/cell-phone-addiction/.

19   Jean Twenge, *iGen. Why Today's Super Connected Kids Are Growing Up Less Rebellious, More Tolerant, Less Happy, and Completely Unprepared for Adulthood* (New York: Atria Books, 2018).

staring at your screen . . . I've had to pinch myself to see if I'm dreaming—and believe me, I want to be dreaming, because ever since we met, something seems to be messing with my sleep.[20]

Speaking of sleep—sleep trouble is a common problem among those struggling with mental illness. Mental illness often causes sleep disturbance, and sleep disturbances often exacerbate mental health struggles. In a 2020 report, the Center for Disease Control (CDC) reported approximately 26 percent of American adults had insufficient sleep, meaning less than an average of seven hours per night; and 77 percent of American high school students reported that, on average, they get less than eight hours of sleep per night.[21]

According to an article by the American Psychological Association, since the COVID-19 pandemic, 66 percent of Americans report sleep-related issues, trouble falling asleep, trouble staying asleep, poor quality of sleep, or sleeping too much (more than nine hours per twenty-four hours).[22] *Sixty-six percent* of Americans have sleep trouble! The article also noted that melatonin sales went up 42 percent in 2020.

While multiple factors contribute to modern sleep issues, too much screen time is recognized as a leading factor. Not only do the blue lights of modern devices confuse our bodies' natural circadian rhythms; but

---

20 Catherine Price, *How to Break Up with Your Phone: The 30-Day Plan to Take Back Your Life* (New York: Ten Speed Press, 2018), vii.

21 "Sleep Health." Centers for Disease Control and Prevention/National Center for Health Statistics, last reviewed February 23, 2023,https://www.cdc.gov/nchs/fastats/sleep-health.htm.

22 Zara Abrams, "Growing Concerns About Sleep," *American Psychological Association,* June 1, 2021, https://www.apa.org/monitor/2021/06/news-concerns-sleep#:~:text=Since%20the%20pandemic%20began%2C%20researchers,in%20America%202021%2C%20APA.

thirty seconds of media of any kind gives dozens of images, words, and ideas for our brain to process and make sense of as we attempt to drift off to sleep.

Stimulation can be defined as "to excite to greater activity" or "to arouse" the body and mind.[23] The ability to be raised to excitement or to be aroused is not a bad thing in and of itself. I am not suggesting that we all need to be monks in rural Thailand who never watch anything moving faster than a jumping cricket. (I do not know if they have crickets in Thailand, but you get the point.) That's not the world many of us live in. And I am grateful.

I am grateful that I have access to so much information. I love that I can wonder if Thailand has crickets and know the answer in a matter of seconds. That is really exciting to me. I enjoy a good YouTube channel as much as the next person. But from what I have noticed in my own life and the lives of my clients, we are too stimulated. Most things in excessive amounts can be dangerous. I think many of our mental health struggles, including anxiety, depression, anger, attention difficulties, memory issues, and addictive behaviors are aggravated by overstimulation. Our brains were not created to consume so much information so rapidly, so continuously, and in such copious amounts.

And it is not just the amount of time. I used to tell my husband, "I'm not on Facebook that much." It was true. I put time restrictions on my social media. I spent less than ten minutes on social media a day. But one day, it hit me. It is not only the amount of time that matters. It is the amount of stimulation. In approximately thirty seconds of

---

23 "Stimulation," Merriam Webster Dictionary, 2024, https://www.merriam-webster.com/dictionary/stimulation.

scrolling, I was exposed to at least ten to fifteen different posts, images, video shorts, and stupid comments from people who clearly do not know what they are talking about, not to mention that cute dress on the sidebar. (I still want that dress, by the way.) I felt excitement; I smiled at a photo of my niece; I rolled my eyes at that comment; I missed my friend in another state; and I coveted that dress. That is a lot of mental activity—and it was crammed into thirty seconds, so it didn't even occur to me that I was over stimulated.

In recent years, I have become familiar with the term Highly Sensitive Person (HSP). I know some of you are rolling your eyes or chuckling right now. I see you! You are probably not an HSP then. That is okay. Jesus still loves you. Haha. Anyway, highly sensitive persons are people who are—hang on to your seat—highly sensitive. Not just emotionally sensitive like many of you are thinking. It really refers to people who are more sensitive to stimulation: sights, sounds, smells, tastes, and physical sensations.

According to Elaine Aron's book, *The Highly Sensitive Person*, HSPs make up approximately 15 to 20 percent of the population.[24] That is quite a few of us. The point is that for those of us who are highly sensitive, overstimulation is even more dangerous to our mental health. While some may be able to handle several minutes per day on the internet, some of us have to be even more careful.

The technological age does not just offer too much *stimulation*. It is too much *information*. We hear about top executives in Washington, our old college roommate's mother-in-law's cat, a Burmese refugee family in Europe, tribal warfare in Sudan, and thousands of other stories in

---

24   Elaine Aron, *The Highly Sensitive Person: How to Thrive When the World Overwhelms You* (New York: Broadway Books, 1996).

the span of *seconds*. We are not created to handle so much information—to know everything. And we do not need to. All we need to know is that which God is calling us to today. "'Sufficient for the day is its own trouble,'" Jesus said.[25]

When we slow down enough to identify what is actually stressing us out; causing us anxiety; and making us feel hopeless, helpless, and frustrated with life, we can come upon some interesting insights. How much of our mental and emotional distress is related to our actual lives? How much of our emotional distress is about the people we actually do life with and are responsible for: our immediate families, local communities, coworkers, or ourselves? There is plenty there to weigh most of us down and to cause concern. Some of that is unavoidable. Life is hard. Until Jesus returns, we will have trouble.

However, what I have found is that there is this other stuff that weighs us down—that subconscious matter that we cannot always put our finger on but that's there swirling in the back of our heads—the call to prayer for a missing six-year-old boy, for that coworker's mother's recent cancer diagnosis, for the Christian church in northern India whose building has been burned down by extremists. I'm just highlighting Christian communities here. Consider the other "regular" news—tsunami in a South Pacific Island you've never heard of, the stock market numbers, the school shooting in an adjacent state. How does one absorb this?

Many of us are so accustomed to this deluge of information, we do not even think twice about it. We may see ourselves as desensitized, numb, or invulnerable. I have heard people flat out tell me it does not

---

25   Matthew 6:34

affect them. They can handle it. If this is you, I am happy for you—also, I am not sure I believe you.

Okay, maybe you really do feel like you can handle it, and maybe you can. But when clients who come in with incredible amounts of anxiety, cannot sleep at night, and were recently diagnosed with high blood pressure tell me their media consumption doesn't affect these things, it takes everything in me not to raise an eyebrow. I am fully aware that there are many factors that contribute to a person's level of anxiety or depression, just like there are many factors that can contribute to physical health. But what we consume is one of those factors to consider. To ignore our mental and emotional consumption is not a good idea. Your emotional metabolism may be able to handle more than someone else, but I think it is still a factor. Phew, all of that is heavy, I know. Good news—there are things we can do about it, and there is a small army of people who are on the journey to protecting themselves and their children from the danger of overstimulation.

BIBLICAL PERSPECTIVE

What is the antidote to overstimulation? Two words come to mind: *guard and focus*. "Keep your heart with all vigilance, for from it flow the springs of life" (Prov. 4:23). We all have a responsibility to guard our hearts and minds—to care for this beautiful soul God created and gave His life for. And we must also be focused as Jesus was when He walked the earth. He was intentional, undistracted, and unwavering in His mission from the Father.

I think we are called to the same. So many things are vying for our attention, but we are called to guard our hearts and focus on the work

God has called us to—the work of turning the majority of our time and attention (our mental capacities) on the people, places, and things that our Lord has called us to. That is a vague, but important, concept, which I will explore with more practical thoughts below.

REDUCE EXPOSURE

For many, this will take intentional discipline. Reduce the amount of exposure to screens—particularly the internet—and even more specifically, social media. I highly recommend silencing all social media notifications. Social media outlets include Facebook, Instagram, X, TikTok, Snapchat, YouTube, Discord, LinkedIn, Pinterest, and Reddit—to name a few. These platforms provide a lot of mental exposure. It is like a UV ray one thousand for your brain. In a one-minute scroll, you can be exposed to dozens of posts, images, advertisements, and comments from a number of different people. Multiply that by fifty-eight times a day—it is a lot of stimulation.

I am not saying you have to get rid of it altogether, although some of the most peaceful, present, emotionally healthy people I know spend very little time on it. I would highly recommend a social media detox for at least thirty days. You may choose to completely or almost completely remove social media from your daily life. For any media use, ask yourself, "How can I appreciate this technology and get it to work for me rather than be controlled or harmed by it?" I highly recommend reading *Digital Minimalism* or *How to Break Up with Your Phone* for help with detoxing from screens and turning a new page in relation to your phone.

Consider the following questions before using social media in particular:

- What has my day been like so far?
- How stressed or hurried have I been by work and family demands?

Many people go to the internet and social media to "wind down"; but I am telling you, it doesn't work. It feels like it will satisfy, and it does satisfy some things; but for many people (especially those struggling with anxiety, depression, anger, or loneliness), social media is a danger, not a solution. Most people end up feeling more anxious, more depressed, angrier, and lonelier—not less—after using social media.

RESIST THE URGE TO CHECK YOUR PHONE

Every time you look at your phone, you are mentally leaving the place you currently are and the thing you were focusing on (work, your kids, your housework, your meal). When you hear it ping, take a breath and intentionally keep doing what you were doing for at least a minute or two. *You should be under no obligation to answer a text or email within two minutes.* Okay, maybe there is an exception if you are an on-duty EMS worker. Maybe. I have sat with teenagers who believe they will absolutely lose their chances of social success forever if they do not respond to their classmate immediately. To their credit, this may be true of some friends; but in that case, we have some other problems (more on this later). If the thing that is happening on the phone (a text conversation with a friend, for example) is important to you and you want to respond promptly, try stopping what you are doing and just take a few minutes to focus on that text conversation. Better yet, call the person, if possible, and have a present and focused conversation.

Some of you have your mouth open right now—did she just say *call* them? If possible, yes. Now that we are slowing down and not being so hurried all the time (We are, right?), you have time to chat with your friend on the phone or keep texting in an intentional way, if that's what you prefer.

Respect Other People's Right to Not Have to Be Glued to Their Devices

Give your loved ones, friends, and employees permission to be present in their day and not need to respond to your text, email, or Snapchat immediately. I have heard young people be extremely hurt or offended because their friend did not text them back. When I ask how long ago they reached out to this friend, they say things like "last night" or "four hours ago." I'm not naïve to the fact that for most young people, a non-immediate response may very well be a rejection. I am just arguing that it should not be! Give your friends time to think, reflect, and respond well when they have a good chance to. You would benefit from this gift from your friends, so give it to them as well. Let them know they do not have to respond immediately.

Have a Designated Place for Your Phone in Your Home and Leave It There

You do not have to have it with you at all times. It is not an appendage. Contrary to popular belief, it is possible to go to the bathroom without a phone (preaching to myself). Having distance from your phone helps remove the temptation to fill spare moments with things you really do not need, like looking at the current weather in Siberia.

CHOOSE RESTAURANTS THAT DO NOT HAVE TVS PLAYING

My husband once counted how many TVs were playing at a restaurant we ate at. There were *forty-two*! I am not even joking. It is hard to listen to your spouse or truly enjoy your meal when American crime shows are playing on screens every direction you look. If you really like the restaurant for other reasons, see if they have an outside patio or pick up takeout and go to the park.

AVOID HAVING MORE THAN ONE SCREEN GOING ON AT ONE TIME

If you are working on the computer, do not play a YouTube video on your phone at the same time. If a family member is playing a video game, do not catch up on videos from your social media feed in the same room. Guard your heart and mind. No one else will take responsibility for safeguarding your mind against too much stimulation. It is our responsibility to do this for ourselves—and our children, too.

Speaking of children, parents often ask me how they get their kids to acquire a healthier habit: trying a new skill, spending more time with friends, enjoying less screen time, or being open and transparent. My response is usually the same—focus on yourself first. Kids are not stupid. They can see right through our pretense. If you are telling the kid who you love that they should do something, have a good honest look at yourself and see if there are improvements you need to make in your own life.

I am not saying you need to be perfect in order to give your kids direction or set limits. There is definitely a place for specific strategies for managing screen time with children. I am just choosing not to focus on that in this book. My main advice here is to live out what you say you value. Show your kids a better way.

CONSIDER PRACTICING SOME SCREEN SABBATHS

Utilize the *do not disturb* features on your phone. It could be thirty minutes over lunch break, a couple of hours in an afternoon, or even an entire day if possible. If the matter is urgent and someone really needs to reach you, usually multiple calls from the same number will come through. Also, many of us are around other people with phones on. If someone really needs to reach you, they can probably find a way, too. There is an element of rest and trust here. What did followers of Jesus do for two thousand years before they had cell phones?

ASK YOURSELF WHY YOU ARE DRAWN TO NEEDING TO BE DISTRACTED SO MUCH

We are not going for critical, self-condemning shame here. Take a curious approach and ask yourself, *What am I trying to escape from right now?* Are there other ways—healthier ways or just a variety of ways—that I can cope with whatever I am feeling (be it boredom, tiredness, or loneliness)?

PRACTICE THE FORTY-EIGHT-HOUR RULE OR SIMILAR MINIMALIST STRATEGY

When you see something you want, choose to wait at least forty-eight hours before you purchase it. Take that time to consider your motivation for buying this thing and if it is in line with the person you want to be.

ENGAGE IN PHYSICAL ACTIVITIES TO WIND DOWN, RATHER THAN TURNING TO MEDIA

Cal Newport suggests this strategy in his book, *Digital Minimalism.* Go for a walk or a run without music playing or your Apple watch constantly giving your vital signs. Newport also suggests practicing the art of being alone.[26] Solitude is a lost practice in our modern world, but Jesus practiced it a lot. Being alone can be quite overwhelming for a lot of people. Many do not like being alone with their thoughts and feelings. If this is you, ask yourself why. What are you mentally running from?

I can empathize with how difficult it can be to face one's own thoughts, but not doing so over a long period of time can be dangerous. Consider journaling, praying, or talking with a trusted friend or professional counselor about the thoughts and feelings that overwhelm you. Sometimes just naming the thoughts out loud can help.

SCHEDULE AND PLACE LIMITS ON "LOW QUALITY LEISURE"[27]

Newport also suggests scheduling specific days and times in your week that you engage in various media outlets. For example, Newport commends one digital minimalist (those who take an offensive approach to guarding their time and attention when it comes to media

---

26   Cal Newport, *Digital Minimalism: Choosing a Focused Life in a Noisy World* (New York: Penguin Random House, 2019).
27   Cal Newport, *Digital Minimalism: Choosing a Focused Life in a Noisy World* (New York: Penguin Random House, 2019).

use) who told the people in his life that he would be available to talk on the phone every workday on his drive home. Rather than spend a lot of time texting and commenting on friend's social media posts, he wanted to prioritize meaningful conversations on a regular basis. John Mark Comer (author of *The Elimination of Hurry* previously mentioned) talks about setting aside a block of time once a week in which he checks email and social media.[28]

EMBRACE THE AWKWARDNESS OF NOT BEING ON YOUR PHONE IN PUBLIC PLACES

Many of us are frequently on our phone simply because we are uncomfortable without them. Anybody else—or is it just me who feels so incredibly awkward waiting in the dentist's office just looking around? At least for those under forty, this feels weird. When I started practicing being present and unhurried, people noticed and looked confused. *Why are you just standing there smiling at me in this grocery store checkout line? Don't you have a phone or something?* I was sure they were thinking this as they peered at me from the corner of their eye and then looked right back to their phones when my eyes met theirs.

Be prepared, young people especially, if you stop looking at your phone all the time, you may find that people notice you. I have had people come to me and ask if I was all right because I was just existing somewhere, instead of looking busy or distracted on my phone. Good news—awkwardness is survivable (more on that in the "pressure to maintain an image" chapter).

---

28   John Mark Comer, *The Ruthless Elimination of Hurry* (Colorado Springs: Water-Brook, 2019).

Identify Your Motivation

Why do you want to reduce stimulation? Why is this important to you? Are you struggling with anxiety, depression, anger, memory issues, or headaches? Are you curious about whether reducing your stimulation could be helpful to you? Do you want to spend more time being present with your kids or friends? This leads into one of the most important paragraphs of this book.

Identify Your Priorities

Picture yourself years from now, toward the end of your life. How would you have wanted your younger self to spend your time and your mental and emotional energy? What work, hobbies, and endeavors do you want to engage in regularly? What people do you want to spend the most time with? What do you want your mind to be filled with much of the time? Everyone will have normal life stressors—many of those things are not avoidable—but some mental stress and mental clutter is avoidable if we take the responsibility to guard our minds. This quote from Cal Newport really resonates with me: "You only have so much time and mental space. How do you want to fill it?"[29]

Have these priorities in mind if you choose to reduce your mental clutter. You are going to need them because I think you will find you actually have so much time and mental space. Many people go to their phones or check their email out of habit. They do not even think about it. Whenever we have a free moment literally anywhere, what do most people do? Get out their phones. We fill our heads with clutter—mental junk that wears at our souls. Take the challenge. When you stop

---

29   Cal Newport, *Digital Minimalism: Choosing a Focused Life in a Noisy World* (New York: Penguin Random House, 2019).

exposing yourself to so much clutter, you will not know what to do with yourself. So have some ideas ready.

What interests have you wanted to pursue but you have always told yourself you don't have time? Is it gardening, fishing, taking your dog for an evening walk, baking bread, tinkering with cars, painting your bathroom, building model planes with your grandson, star gazing for a few minutes before bed, enjoying candlelit baths with your spouse—what is it? You will find yourself less hurried as you make and embrace more spare moments. Are you making dinner and feeling that pull to see what everyone else in the world is doing? Stop. Instead, just open the window and let some fresh air in while you sneak a small piece of pre-dinner chocolate and savor the bite.

Think of people you promised to pray for and *actually* pray for them. When I stopped opening my phone every spare moment, I was shocked how much time, energy, and mental space I actually had. Do I always take advantage of it? No, I am human, too. But when I do take the time to engage in the things that are important to me (that I used to say I did not have time for), it had wondrous effects on my mental health, relationships, and finances.

So the next time you have a spare moment (you will find you have a lot of them as you practice unhurriedness), resist the urge to open your phone. See if you can resist the urge to even hold it and look at the message on the lock screen (we have all done that). You are not a slave to that device! We have not reached the AI (artificial intelligence) apocalypse just yet; so take a deep breath, look around, and think about those priorities you identified. What from that list could you engage in right now? You probably only have a few minutes—maybe even seconds—but what kinds of things would you do if you were the kind of person who lived what they said was important to them?

REFLECTIVE QUESTIONS:

1. Do you agree that overstimulation is a problem for our culture?

2. Do you often feel like your mind is cluttered or filled with too many thoughts or images? Do you often notice yourself bothered by a post or comment you saw on social media?

3. Do you frequently experience symptoms such as headaches, muscle tension, blurred vision, high blood pressure, sleep trouble, stress eating, trouble concentrating, or memory trouble?

4. Do you often feel frazzled even though things in your life are going okay at the moment?

5. Are there any areas of your life that you believe you guard your mind well? What helps you to be able to do that?

6. Do you know anyone who seems peaceful much of the time? Why do you think that is?

7. What hesitations or objections do you have to reduce your stimulation exposure?

8. What is one small (or large) step you could take to practice guarding your heart and mind from too much stimulation?

RECOMMENDED RESOURCES:

- *Digital Minimalism* by Cal Newport
- *How to Break Up with Your Phone* by Catherine Price

CHAPTER 3

Danger Three: Pressure to Maintain an Image

"There are more things ... likely to frighten us than there are to crush us.
We suffer more in imagination than in reality."[30]

—Seneca (Rome 20-60 AD)

A friend of ours recently asked my husband (who is in the science and technology field) if he thought that AI would ever be a threat to humans. For example, could machines ever get so advanced that they could outsmart humans and harm them? My husband's response was insightful. He said that in a way, we are allowing technology to take over our lives already. What is scary is that technology dictates what we think about; how we think; what we like or do not like; who we associate with; and how we spend our time, affections, and money. But AI did not create this. We did. And we participate in unhealthy practices that reveal the weakest parts of ourselves: our pride, our insecurities, and our desire to feel in control.

---

30   "Dealing with Stress: 12 Proven Strategies for Stress Relief from Stoicism," Daily Stoic: Ancient Wisdom for Everyday Life, last updated 2021, https://www.dailys-toic.com/stress-relief.

The Problem

There is this phenomenon I have seen among young people—this feeling of immense dissatisfaction with themselves. They have a hard time finding motivation for life, are seemingly disappointed in what they have accomplished so far, and have dim views of what they could accomplish in the future. When I ask what they are interested in, they struggle to identify much. And the thing they are interested in, they feel unsure that they could make a living off of it and question if they are really even good at it.

"I'd like to _____, but I'm not nearly good enough to make it in that."

"I don't know what I bring to the world."

"If I can't do anything great, I don't even know why I'm here."

"I'm not sure my life is worth living; I just don't see the point."

Of course, not every young person shares this way of thinking, but it is a pattern with many. And while it may not originate with clinical depression, it can certainly lead there.

I call this phenomenon the "superhero syndrome." It is this idea that unless one is literally saving the universe in some unique way, then it's appropriate to question that life may not be worth living. In the information age, where a person has access to unlimited information, resources, and opportunities, many of us feel immense pressure to do "something great" with our lives. But young people can feel this pressure on an exponential level. Teens and college students have expressed to me great anxiety about the future. They worry that they do not measure up, that they are just not enough, that they are not interesting enough to have friends or find a partner. Young people talk about doing something that will put them in the history books and maybe bring their followers up to two million; or else, what is the point?

Cal Newport notes that social media provides a breeding ground for intermittent positive reinforcement and exploits the human need to be socially acceptable.[31] Every time we get a notification that someone "likes" our post, we get rewarded with feel-good hormones that make us feel seen and affirmed. But this reward is intermittent, meaning that we never know if we will get the social approval or not. We are painfully aware that we may not get the response we want. Someone may leave an unfavorable comment or the "angry face" emotion, or even worse: after three days, no one besides our grandmother liked our post. And that is not even mentioning the anxiety of what other people may post about you! You never know who could be taking a video of you; and before school starts the next day, half your class has seen an awkward picture of you eating a sandwich. The pressure can leave many people completely preoccupied and stressed out about protecting their online image.

In her book about the "iGen" generation (those born between 1995 and 2022), Jean Twenge points out that iGeners are very concerned about "emotional safety," maybe even as much as physical safety. "This is a fascinating, perhaps distinctly iGen idea: the world is an inherently dangerous place because every social interaction carries the risk of being hurt. You never know what someone is going to say, and there's no way to protect yourself from it."[32] Twenge goes on to present research demonstrating an increase in anxiety, depression, and loneliness among iGen that is closely linked to widespread smart phone use.

---

31   Cal Newport, *Digital Minimalism: Choosing a Focused Life in a Noisy World* (New York: Penguin Random House, 2019), 17.

32   Jean Twenge, *iGen. Why Today's Super Connected Kids Are Growing Up Less Rebellious, More Tolerant, Less Happy, and Completely Unprepared for Adulthood* (New York: Atria Books, 2018), 157.

I struggled to identify an accurate name for this chapter and to describe this particular danger to mental health. It encompasses several different ideas that, in my best attempts, I have entitled as pressure to maintain an image. It is this constant push to prove ourselves—to others and to ourselves. I believe this is a cultural value of our time. The message of the world is, "Work intently at finding and creating your own image—your persona, your aesthetic, your vibe, your higher self. Then you must religiously obey the image you have created. Be true to it. Make it clear to others. Express yourself to the world. Be loud and proud about who you are."

But this is a distorted view. We are created in the image of God.[33] Our deepest meaning, purpose, and identity rest securely in our Creator. Our purpose is to reflect His love to each other and to the world. We build, love, create, think, feel, and speak as a reflection of God's character and for His glory. When we do not remember this, we can become anxiety-ridden that our identity rests on us alone. That is a lot of pressure.

"I know I should go to the group. I think it would be good for me. It's just . . . " My client hesitated, looked at me, and continued, "I guess I just feel behind. Like those women are just so ahead of me. They seem like they have it all together. Here I am over here just trying not to look at porn and get out of this toxic relationship. I thought I was doing well; but when I see those women are struggling with something so small, I feel not enough."

This is not a specific client's story but a representation of many women I have sat with in professional counseling. Many of us can relate to feeling like we have come far in our healing journey but still get hung up on insecurity. The crazy thing is that those people at the

---

33 Genesis 1:27

Bible study, work event, or friend group are probably thinking the same thing about you! That's one of the most insightful things I've learned as a professional counselor—the realization that no one is exempt from struggle, and everyone feels some insecurity about some area of their life. People have problems. It is a part of being human. Anyone who says they have it all together does not. Period.

My kids brought home a book from the library entitled *Joan Proctor: Dragon Doctor*.[34] It is a true story about a woman born in 1897 who, since childhood, was fascinated by reptiles. She would keep and care for lizards, snakes, and crocodiles. In her late teens, she began working for the Zoological Society of London and gained international acclaim for her work researching, writing papers, caring for the animals, and designing exhibits for them.

As I was reading the book to my kids, I was fascinated by this woman's story. How inspiring to see a woman who knew what she was passionate about and had unprecedented success as a woman in the early 1900s. I felt myself even a little envious of her. *How lucky she was to have such purpose and passion*, I thought to myself. Then I read the more detailed biography at the back of the book and was stunned. Joan Proctor died at thirty-four years old. She suffered from chronic intestinal illness since childhood; she never went to college, and she never was married or had children.[35] Her story struck me forcefully. Here I was envious of someone who died younger than I was at the time I read the book to my two sons. It brought me great perspective. No one has a perfect life, and everyone has something to be grateful for.

---

34   Patricia Valdez, *Joan Proctor, Dragon Doctor: The Woman Who Loved Reptiles* (New York: Random House Children's Books, 2018).

35   "Happy Birthday Joan Proctor," Zoological Society of London, August 4, 2017, https://www.zsl.org/news-and-events/news/happy-birthday-joan-procter.

Comparison has always been a problem. The first temptation was literally, "You will be like God."[36] And then shortly after that, a sibling jealousy ended in murder.[37] But today, I believe that there is even more danger to our mental health through comparison. Because of globalization and the internet, we are bombarded with too many options and too many opportunities, which can lead to a sense of overwhelm and decision fatigue. We are exposed daily to carefully crafted images of people who we barely know or do not really know at all. Social media constantly shows us people who are "winning" at bread-making, composting, homeschooling, house-flipping, car-fixing, wardrobe-perfecting, and on and on. We can feel chronically behind, like our little lives are sad and pathetic when everyone else out there is living their best life.

Here I go folding another load of laundry and praying that I can make it to the bedroom before my toddler smears his chocolate-covered hands all over the clean clothes . . . I'm probably a bad mom for giving him chocolate in the first place. When the sky is the limit, when there is nothing standing in our way except ourselves, we can become anxiety-ridden. *The only reason I am not that guy with the private jet is because either I am somehow falling short or others are to blame—society, the government—you pick.*

Earlier this year, a movie came out; and for a few weeks, everyone seemed to be talking about it. Several of my female clients deeply resonated with one quote in particular: "It is literally impossible to be a woman . . . we have to be extraordinary, but somehow we're always doing it wrong."[38] The quote goes on to describe the impossible societal

---

36   Genesis 3:5
37   Genesis 4
38   Yvonne Villarreal, "Read the Stirring Monologue about Womanhood America Ferrera delivers in 'Barbie,'" *Los Angeles Times*, July 23, 2023, https://www.latimes.com/entertainment-arts/movies/story/2023-07-23/barbie-america-ferrera-monologue.

expectations placed upon women. While it is true that there have been society factors that put pressures on women which are both unfair and even cruel, it is impossible and unwise to ignore the question of how much pressure we have placed on ourselves. I may not have put it there to start with, but I have to ask myself: do I keep it there?

Do I play the game—that competition game that says I must dress my kids in trendy clothes, look attractive but not too sensual, and only host people in my house if it is well-designed and put together? It makes me wonder: is society holding me to impossible standards, or am I? Let us take it step further: society *is* holding me to an impossible standard, but why am I? This pressure to create and maintain an image is extremely stressful for many people; and for some, the pressure leads to despairing of life itself. But do we really have no other choice? I believe we do.

If you do not like the game, stop playing it. Stop dying your gray hair, volunteering for every event at your kid's school, and only posting filtered pictures of yourself from weird angles—unless you actually just want to! There is nothing wrong with those things. My point is, we unnecessarily stress ourselves, draining our time and money on things that we do not actually value. We need to ask ourselves, "Would I actually suffer any negative consequences (lose my job or a relationship) if I did not hold myself to such unrealistic standards? Would anyone actually even notice or care if I stopped trying so hard to pretend to have it all together? And if I did lose those things, are they worth it? Are they worth my mental health and the health of those closest to me?"

I can hear some of you saying right now, "But I don't really struggle with that. I don't care about what anyone else does. I do me." I know some of you are thinking this because I've thought it, too! Who wants to admit they are a copycat—a "follower"? We are Americans, after all! We are fiercely independent at our core. But speaking as a woman in particular, we struggle with this. It can change over time and through different seasons. When you are twelve and heading to your first day of seventh grade, what is on your mind? *How do I compare? How do I measure up against my peers? Please, God, don't let Johnny notice my pimples today.*

Fast forward a decade or two, and what do I hear from new moms? *I feel like I'm failing. Is breastfeeding this hard for everyone? What is wrong with me?* Fast forward another decade or two. A middle-aged woman, fresh to the empty nest, finds she has no idea what to do with herself. I ask her to describe more of what she feels, and it is something like competition. *Other women seem to have career plans they can't wait to get back to or an exhilarating trip to Israel or an Alaskan cruise. What about me?*

I know this chapter may resonate a little more to the female readers, but men struggle with this, too—just maybe in a different form. For men, it may look like pressure to build a career and amass financial wealth or status symbols such as vehicles or an impressive investment portfolio.

Note: Comparing ourselves to others may not always be bad. Sometimes we look to identify with others for a sense of comfort and connection, to know that we are not alone in our feelings, our struggles, or our sufferings. Sometimes, comparing ourselves to someone else's situation may help us be more grateful or give us a different perspective. But those positive experiences usually come out of strong interpersonal connections with close family and friends who show genuine interest in us. Rarely do we get this sense of connection from the internet; and if we do, it is often not worth all the other negative effects that came with it.

BIBLICAL PERSPECTIVE

Do we ever see Jesus getting sidetracked by comparison? Do we see Him looking at His cousin John and wondering if He is doing better or worse than him? Do we find Jesus irritated that other rabbis had more followers, better pay, or invitations from higher officials? When He gave a hard speech and many of the disciples turned away, did He question whether He was as good as those other preachers? No, He was secure in His identity with His Father. He looked to Him for validation and security. Sure, it's nice to get validation from other people; but at the end of the day, Jesus "did not entrust Himself to them, because He knew all people and needed no one to bear witness about man, for He himself knew what was in man."[39]

He knew that people have their own insecurities, that they were not the best judges of what mattered most. And so, His identity was not dependent on how people saw Him.

The problem is not so much the act of observing yourself against other individuals but in assigning value to yourself based on how you stand beside other people. Whether you feel you are not as good as someone else or that you are better than someone else, the result is the same problem. Pride and self-deprecation are both centered on the self and put men and women as judges. But only God has the authority and the wisdom to assign worth to a human being.

The antidote to comparison is *security*, to be untroubled and steady. It is in knowing who you are, primarily in Christ. We have other

---

39 John 2:24-25

identities, and they do matter (spouse, parent, coworker, citizen, our passions, hobbies, and abilities). We can look to others for motivation and inspiration. But ultimately, our identity and security come from the One Who created us, redeemed us, made a way for us to come back to Him, Who loves us unconditionally, and promises us a home with Him for all time. Therefore, His opinion—what He thinks of us—should be where our eyes focus.

This is where I challenge you to consider why it matters what anyone else is doing. How do you know you are not making the most of your life? Again, as a goal-oriented, dream-big kind of girl, I am not saying just sit and do not aspire to do anything with your life. I am saying, who are you asking first? Whose opinion of how you are doing fills your head? What does the Lord have for you? That is where you want to be, friend. Right there. In the center of His will for you.

Address pride in your heart. Life is not a competition. It is a race but not a competition against others.[40] When Jesus was revealing to Simon Peter a glimpse into what would happen to Him in the future, Peter's question was the classic "What about him?" while nodding his head in John's direction. Jesus said to Peter, "If it is my will that he remain until I come, what is that to you? You follow me!"[41] This interaction has convicted me more than once. It is very easy for us to compare, compete, or make sure others do not have it better than us. I want justice as long as it benefits me, and I want mercy as long as it benefits me.

The parable of the vineyards is another very convicting story that has struck me since childhood. In the parable of the vineyards, Jesus tells the story of a vineyard owner who hires out servants throughout

---

40   2 Timothy 4:7-8; Hebrews 12:1-2
41   John 21:20-22

a long workday. At the end of the day, the workers who started late in the day received the same amount as the workers who started at the beginning of the day. The early workers were disgruntled at what they perceived as injustice. But the vineyard owner (representing God) corrects the early workers by explaining to them that they received exactly what they were promised and to mind their own business. If the owner wants to be generous, why do they care?[42]

As a follower of Jesus, there is no need to prove ourselves. The Word of God makes it clear that you and I are not good enough.[43] We are not—not good enough, not worthy, not up to par—but that is why we need Jesus! Author Dane Orthlund puts it this way: "We cannot present a reason for Christ to finally close off His heart to His own sheep. No such reason exists. Every human friend has a limit . . . With Christ, our sins and weaknesses are the very resume items that qualify us to approach Him."[44] We can rest. We can let go of the need to protect our reputation. We have a responsibility to be genuine, confess, repent, and receive forgiveness; but there is no need to try to prove anything.

"As long as you fix your attention on your sin, you will fail to see how you can be safe. But as long as you look to the high priest [Jesus], you will fail to see how you can be in danger."[45]

What would it be like if people knew you did not have it all together? What if you admitted that openly and did not have to keep up the façade anymore? Somewhere between pride—*I am better than*

---

42   Matthew 20:1-16
43   Romans 3:23
44   Dane Orthlund, *Gentle & Lowly: The Heart of Christ for Sinners and Sufferers* (Wheaton, IL: Crossway, 2020).
45   Orthlund, *Gentle & Lowly*.

other people—and self-deprecation—*I am worse than everyone else*— is the reality. Mental and spiritual health is about seeing ourselves accurately—very flawed and very loved. Friend, there is immense freedom in this. Imagine what it would be like if you did not make decisions based on what others thought of you. What if you could choose a vocation, hobby, friend, buying habits—everything— because it was the right thing to do, because you wanted to, because the people who really matter in your life agree with you, and because the people whose opinion shouldn't matter (acquaintances, celebrities, influencers) didn't.

Being a counselor has helped me feel so connected to humanity. When you repeatedly hear people struggling with the same kinds of things, you begin to realize how similar our experiences are. This gives me so much courage to be vulnerable, to be secure, to let go of comparison and competition because I am mindful of the fact that no one has it all together. Everyone has been low or will feel low at some point in their lives. Here are some things we can try:

GROUND YOURSELF IN THE PROMISES AND HEART OF GOD

In her book, *Unseen: The Gift of Being Hidden in a World that Loves to Be Noticed*, Sara Hagerty challenges us to consider Psalm 139. She reflects on how before we were seen by human eyes, we were seen by God. We were known in secret, hidden from the world but known by God—loved and cherished before we ever had a chance to prove our worth. "My frame was not hidden from you, when I was being made in secret, intricately woven in the depths of the earth. Your eyes saw my unformed substance; in your book were written, every one of them, the days that were formed for me, when as yet there was none of them."[46]Sara continues by highlighting Paul's words. "For you have died, and your life is hidden with Christ in God."[47]

As her subtitle alludes to, the world loves to be noticed; we want to be recognized for our achievements, status updates, and our emotional highs. But there is great comfort and freedom in resting in hiddenness in Christ, knowing that we are intimately loved by One Who sees us when others don't.[48]

ACCEPT AND UTILIZE THE GIFT OF REPENTANCE

Repentance is a gift in that God makes a very simple and clear way for us to handle guilt and shame—confess and repent. "If we confess our sins, He is faithful and just to forgive us our sins and to cleanse us from all unrighteousness."[49] That is an incredible promise which brings so much comfort and security! Knowing that God, the Judge of all the earth, says we can be forgiven if only we ask Him. What is there to hide? This provides much freedom to be open about our struggles and imperfections because we are secure in God's promise to not condemn us or put us to shame. "Indeed, none who wait for you shall be put to shame."[50]

CHOOSE AUTHENTICITY AND VULNERABILITY

By authenticity, I mean actually being what you claim to be. By vulnerability, I mean choosing to be authentic about yourself with other people, even if there is a possibility of being harmed emotionally.

---

46 Psalm 139:15-16
47 Colossians 3:3
48 Sara Hagerty, *Unseen: The Gift of Being Hidden in a World that Loves to Be Noticed* (Grand Rapids, MI: Zondervan, 2017).
49 1 John 1:9
50 Psalm 25:3

There is a lot of confusion and misrepresentation of these two ideas. By authentic and vulnerable, I do *not* mean say whatever you think or feel at all times, even if it is mean, inappropriate, or hurtful. That is not likely to make you or anyone around you feel more secure and less stressed. Vulnerability is not over-sharing, sharing inappropriately, or showing off at how "open book" you are about your problems.

Vulnerability is about being a person who aligns with what you say you value—the person you would like to be, no matter how others may respond. It takes courage and security to be able to practice this. However, practicing vulnerability and genuineness is crucial if we want to reduce stress, anxiety, depression, and loneliness (more on this in the next chapter). Many of us learned how *not* to be vulnerable in middle school, but those tactics you learned to survive a difficult season will not serve you well if you want to live an emotionally healthy life.

Here are some ways in which one can practice vulnerability:

- Owning and confessing the ways you messed up
- *Not* owning up to things that actually were not your fault
- Owning and accepting that you do not know or aren't competent in something
- Acknowledging your feelings, including insecurities
- Expressing genuine gratitude rather than acting as if you do not need others

Here are some examples that are *not* authentic and vulnerable:

Example 1: Someone in your church small group shares that they had a wisdom tooth taken out this week; and you respond with, "You think that's bad? I had to have three taken out last year!" While it may be true, this is not vulnerable. It comes across as competitive and insecure.

Example 2: You have a hurtful argument with your spouse; and you post on social media, "Ugh. Being married is so hard when you always have to be the bigger person in the relationship. #prayforme" While it is true that this is vulnerable in the sense that it is opening oneself to criticism and being hurt, it is hurtful to expose the spouse in this public way and again feels more about competition and gaining popularity. It is not humble and probably not helpful in getting the kind of help you actually need.

Example 3: You run into someone you know at the grocery store, and she kindly compliments your outfit. You say, "Oh, this old thing? I'm so embarrassed you're even seeing me like this. I usually never wear sweatpants in public!" Your friend is wearing sweatpants, and you know it. This is the opposite of vulnerability; it is comparison, competition, and insecurity and hurtful to the other person.

Some examples of emotionally healthy authenticity and vulnerability:

- Example 1: You run into a difficult situation with a client at work and do not know what to do. You feel embarrassed and incompetent. You take a deep breath; go to your boss; and say, "I feel embarrassed asking you about this, but I really don't know what to do. Would you be willing to help me?"
- Example 2: You hurt your friend's feelings, and an apology would be in order. You go to her and say, "I am genuinely sorry for what I said last night. Would you forgive me?"

- Example 3: Your spouse says something hurtful to you. Instead of defending yourself, saying something hurtful in return, or throwing a hair dryer at them, you simply say, "Ouch."
- Example 4: You are with a group of your buddies. A few of them start talking about a topic you do not know much about, and they ask what you think. Instead of acting like you know what you are talking about or cracking a joke to divert attention, you simply say, "I actually don't know enough about this topic to have an opinion on it yet, but I'm enjoying hearing what you guys think."
- Example 5: You share with your men's group at church, "It's so hard for me to say this, but my marriage is in a really rough spot. My wife told me last night that she wants to separate. I'm terrified, and I don't know what to do. I need help."

It's like the well-circulated meme that says:

"The three hardest things to say are:
I was wrong,
I need help,
Worcestershire sauce."[51]

---

51   I have no idea who to cite as the original author of this meme content; but if you are out there and read this, thank you.

In *Daring Greatly*, author Brené Brown points out that we tend to see vulnerability in ourselves as a negative thing, something we should feel ashamed of.[52] But when we see other people being vulnerable, we see it as a positive thing, something to be admired and appreciated. Then there are people who see vulnerability as a negative thing for everyone. They see vulnerability as a weakness; a chance to get ahead of another person. It is no surprise that these folks often have difficulty in their marriages, work relationships, and friendships.

If you are one of these people or one who struggles to understand and practice healthy vulnerability, consider seeing a licensed professional counselor. An inability to be authentic and vulnerable with trustworthy people can greatly affect your mental health and your relationship to yourself, others, and God. It is worth finding a good therapist who can help you identify and process your life story in order to gain better self-awareness and healthy coping skills.

REMIND YOURSELF THAT MOST THINGS IN LIFE DO NOT NEED TO BE A COMPETITION

Stop competing with your sister-in-law's beautiful sense of style, your coworker's attention from the boss, your friend's kids' behavior, and that guy at your church with the impeccable red mustang with shiny rims. (I really do not know what cars are considered cool these days, so insert whatever makes sense here.)When you feel the temptation to compete with others when it is not necessary, try acknowledging their strengths rather than trying to prove you are better than them.

---

52   Brené Brown, *Daring Greatly: How the Courage to be Vulnerable Transforms the Way We Live, Love, Parent, and Lead* (New York, NY: Gotham Books, 2012).

ALLOW YOURSELF TO CRY

The act of crying can actually be quite healthy.[53] It helps the body process and express sadness and grief.[54] It releases endorphins that help the body regulate and feel better. Expressing our sadness through tears can build healthy connections with other people. Excessive or frequent crying may be a sign that you should seek professional help, but crying is a symptom, not the problem itself. And yes, both men and women can and should cry if they feel the need to. Crying as a way to express feelings is a preventative action one can take in managing stress and preventing anxiety and depression. Not being able to cry may be a sign to seek professional help.

REDUCE SOCIAL MEDIA CONSUMPTION

If you are struggling with unhappiness, depression, anger, or anxiety, take an honest look at whether the media you are consuming is contributing to this problem. Jessica Barley, a fellow licensed professional counselor, puts it this way: "I wonder if actually *not* posting—not looking for affirmation from others—could be an act of worship; an act of trust. Trusting that because the Father sees us—we don't always need everyone else to."[55]

---

53 Asmir Gračanin, et al. "Why crying does and sometimes does not seem to alleviate mood: a quasi-experimental study," Motivation and Emotion vol. 39, 6, August 23, 2015,https://doi.org/10.1007/s11031-015-9507-9, 953-960.
54 Leo Newhouse, "Is Crying Good for You," Harvard Health Publishing, March 1, 2021, https://www.health.harvard.edu/blog/is-crying-good-for-you-2021030122020.
55 Jessica Barley, email message to author, January 9, 2024.

Purposely Do Things That Are Not Perfect if You Struggle with Perfectionism

Do things that will "stain" your perfect image. I am not suggesting things outside of your values or beliefs of course, but things like intentionally wearing a mismatched outfit or intentionally leaving one bookshelf undusted just to see what happens. Likely, no one will even much notice or care; and you will help adjust your mindset that you can relax and stop putting so much energy into proving yourself.

Help Cultivate Environments that Encourage Authenticity and Vulnerability

At home, at work, and with friends, compliment and encourage others when you notice something about them. Thank others when you see them putting themselves out there in a genuine way. Make it your practice to refuse to participate in degrading others, gossiping, or insincerely flattering. If you encounter someone who seems embarrassed or in a vulnerable situation, help them be at ease with reassurances that they are not alone and that they are still acceptable to you.

This sounds like things we might teach sixth graders; but truthfully, many of us as adults can be just as hurtful (sometimes unintentionally) as an insecure twelve-year-old. But it is time to grow up, reset our thoughts on our identity in Christ, and cultivate environments of healing and care for our fellow human beings. For followers of Jesus, the call should be nothing less. Jesus never took people's vulnerabilities as an opportunity to elevate Himself or make Himself look good. He met people where they were in their brokenness. May it be true of us as well.

Reflective questions:

1. Do you think there is a pressure to create and maintain an image for ourselves?

2. In what ways or areas of your life do you struggle with pride, insecurity, comparing yourself to others, competing with others, or feeling pressured to hide your flaws?

3. Are there any areas of your life that you feel more secure in? What helps you remain secure?

4. What is one small (or large) step you could take to practice living securely in your identity in Christ?

5. Is the Lord calling you to do something that you have been afraid to do because you are too concerned about how it would affect your reputation?

6. Is there anyone in your life that you can encourage, compliment, or be a safe person who will listen without judgment?

Recommended Resources:

- *Gentle and Lowly* by Dane Orthlund (Christian perspective)
- Psalm 139 by King David (Christian perspective)
- *When People Are Big, and God Is Small* by Edward Welch (Christian perspective)

CHAPTER 4
Danger Four: Loneliness

"When we are fiercely independent and self-sufficient,
our disappointments loom large because we have nothing else to focus on."[56]

—Kevin Walker

I sat across from her, a dark-eyed woman in her thirties. She was from Pakistan and was one of a handful of Muslim women who had joined our free English as a Second Language (ESL) Program. I had been leading the ESL program for a few months as a side ministry while I was in graduate school. She and I had just made plans to meet at her house for tea, and she was so excited.

"I have never had anyone in my home in America," she told me.

"How long have you been here?" I asked.

"Four years," she said sadly.

I asked if she had ever been inside an American home. She shook her head no.

---

56   Kevin Walker, "Reading the Stoics with Millennials," Westmont College, March 2019, https://www.westmont.edu/sites/default/files/users/user551/Walker_0.pdf.

My husband also experienced another enlightening exchange in a Southeastern town. He told me how his college dormmates were having a meeting to establish some ground rules for the dorm. Clean the bathroom, wash your dishes, and keep the coffee table uncluttered were some of the suggested agreements. They came to my husband's quiet and gentle South Indian roommate. He sat up a little taller in his chair and tried to sound stern when it was his turn to state his "rule."

"I would like for us to cook a meal together," he said as firmly as he could. "At least once a week."

That was his rule? Wanting to make a meal together? Awkward silence fell as the others looked at each other and shrugged.

I have had the privilege of working with immigrants at various points in my life, particularly in ESL programs and international student ministries. One of the first things immigrants from non-Western cultures notice about our country is that everyone is so busy, and no one seems to have time or want to make time to hang out on a regular basis. They have shared with me how incredibly odd and shocking it was for them to express a desire to spend time with a new American friend, just to hear that "friend" say something like, "Oh yeah, we should get coffee sometime," but make no effort to actually meet.

One international student explained it this way: "In my country, if I want to talk with my friend, I go to her house. She stops what she was doing, and we make tea and a snack together. We talk for maybe a couple of hours, and I help her if she has something she needs to get done. Here"—gesturing her hand toward the people around us—"if I want to see a friend, I must text her to see when she is available and wait three to four weeks to get maybe one hour on her calendar. How strange," she says.

And she is right.

The Problem

Loneliness is a problem in modern America. Cigna Corporation, Morning Consult reports that in December 2021, 58 percent of U.S. adults were lonely.[57] Some report that loneliness rates may be decreasing from 2021 to 2023, possibly in correspondence with recovery from the COVID-19 pandemic. In 2023, the American Psychological Association and Gallup Poll reported that on average 17 percent of American adults felt lonely the day before. However, the rates of loneliness are still significant, especially for those with lower economic status (63 to 72 percent), racial minorities (68 to 75 percent), the elderly (41 percent), and young adults (79 percent).[58]

Outside of statistical data, many of us have anecdotal knowledge that loneliness is a problem for modern Americans. I often ask clients who they consider a support in their life. It is not rare for people to tell me that they do not have many friends outside of their families or that they do not feel they have enough community support. Some clients I have spoken with could not think of a single person they would feel comfortable calling in the middle of the night if they needed to talk.

---

57   Jessica Beuchler, "The Loneliness Epidemic Persists: A Post-Pandemic Look at the State of Loneliness Among U.S. Adults," The Cigna Group, last updated 2024, https://newsroom.thecignagroup.com/loneliness-epidemic-persists-post-pandemic-look.

58   Tori, Deanglis, "Young Adults Are Still Lonely, But the Rates of Loneliness Are Dropping Overall," America Psychological Association, July 1, 2023, https://www.apa.org/monitor/2023/07/young-adults-lonely-pandemic#:~:text=67%25,with%2032%25%20of%20the%20nonlonely.

Many people, especially those younger than thirty, talk about feeling chronically lonely.

Loneliness is a mental health problem.[59] Loneliness is a risk factor that increases anxiety, depression, substances use, and other addictive behaviors. In contrast, positive relationships and strong support systems are buffers against mental, emotional, behavioral, and spiritual problems. A supportive healthy community is vital to one's physical and mental health. Loneliness and feeling disconnected from other people are dangerous and potentially life-threatening.

One of the things people who are considering suicide will say is, "I can't stop thinking about how if I died tomorrow, I'm not sure one person would really care. I don't think anyone's life would really be any different if I was gone."

Loneliness is an even more serious problem for teens and young adults, as are thoughts of suicide. Many young people feel chronically alone, and a large part of that is due to lack of quality, in-person time spent with peers or, really, anyone. Jean Twenge, in her book about iGen, reports that college students in 2016 spent, on average, seven hours less a week on in-person socializing than college students in the late 1980s.[60] She reports that iGeners are not spending that extra time studying or playing sports; they are spending most of that extra time online—texting, streaming services, watching YouTube videos, and engaging in social media.

A seventeen-year-old client and I were discussing how difficult modern life can be. She said, "I kind of wish I lived in another time . . .

---

59   "How Loneliness Can Impact Your Health." Cleveland Clinic, September 30, 2024, https://health.clevelandclinic.org/what-happens-in-your-body-when-youre-lonely

60   Jean Twenge, *iGen. Why Today's Super Connected Kids Are Growing Up Less Rebellious, More Tolerant, Less Happy, and Completely Unprepared for Adulthood* (New York: Atria Books, 2018),71.

" I thought she was about to say Renaissance Europe or post-World War II in the late 1940s; but she continued, "Like when *Friends* was. When was *Friends?*" It took me a second to register what she was talking about. *Friends?* Oh, the TV show. She was talking about the TV show that aired from 1994 to 2004. She commented on how the friends did not have cell phones, how they actually talked to each other and spent quality time together. It was one of her favorite shows.

This high school senior wished she lived thirty years ago—when our lives were not consumed by internet searches and social media anxieties. So much has changed in one generation, and yet our emotional needs are the same. Just spend any amount of time on a college campus. The majority of students will be looking down at their phone, listening to something playing on their phone, or have their phone in their hands, glancing at it habitually.

Distractions from media are making us lonely, as are the other modern dangers we have been addressing in this book—we are too busy and too independent to want to do the hard work of building relationships. "When we are fiercely independent and self-sufficient, our disappointments loom large because we have nothing else to focus on."[61] In other words, we are self-absorbed as a culture. As we have previously mentioned, we are so preoccupied with maintaining our own image and keeping up our reputation that many of us do not have time or desire to "put another thing on our to do list." I mean, who has time for making friends, anyway?

It is true that relationships are hard work. In many ways, they have always been work. Many great tales—ancient and new—involve

---

61   Kevin Walker, "Reading the Stoics with Millennials," Westmont College, March 2019, https://www.westmont.edu/sites/default/files/users/user551/Walker_0.pdf.

people in relationships, relational conflict, and people developing and maintaining relationships. However, I wonder if relationships today are even harder, require more intentionality, more discipline, and more choice than before.

BIBLICAL PERSPECTIVE

Relationships are important and a central theme of the Christian faith. Before time itself began, God the Father, Son, and Holy Spirit were in community with each other.[62] After time began, God said it was not good for man to be alone, so He created a companion for the first man.[63] When Jesus physically walked the earth in human form, He established and participated in community. He went to synagogue and participated in religious gatherings as we read in Luke 2:41-42: "Now His parents went to Jerusalem every year at the Feast of the Passover. And when He was twelve years old, they went up according to custom."

Likewise, in Luke 4:16 it says, "And He came to Nazareth, where He had been brought up. And as was His custom, He went to the synagogue on the Sabbath day, and He stood up to read." Jesus initiated layers of community and relationships. He chose the twelve disciples as close companions; He chose three of those disciples as His intimate inner circle; and He chose seventy-two followers as His ministry partners.[64]

God called people into community in the Scriptures, and He calls people into community still. Through the New Testament writers, God calls His followers—including future followers—to not neglect meeting with one another, to spur

---

62   John 1:1-3
63   Genesis 2:18
64   Luke 6:12-16, Mark 9:2, Luke 10:1

each other on, and to encourage one another.[65] In the final book of the Bible, God gives us a glimpse into what eternity will be like, and guess what—community will be there. "After this I looked, and behold, a great multitude that no one could number, from every nation, from all tribes and peoples and languages, standing before the throne and before the Lamb, clothed in white robes, with palm branches in their hands, and crying out with a loud voice, 'Salvation belongs to our God who sits on the throne, and to the Lamb!'"[66]

In his book *The Great Divorce*, C.S. Lewis uses imagination and fantastical language to describe what Hell might be like: a dreary, gray city where the inhabitants slowly move farther and farther away from each other.[67] Lewis imagined Hell as:

Forever cut off from God's presence, eternally unable to know God's love and mercy . . . To be totally separated from other creatures, to be wholly and increasingly self-absorbed, makes that self smaller and smaller, and ultimately will result in the person ceasing to be a self. To someone who has been wholly centered on self, having that self cease to exist would be the ultimate possible loss.[68]

Lewis raised an interesting idea—that Hell is about being alone.

---

65 Hebrews. 10:24-25
66 Revelation 7:9-10
67 C.S. Lewis, *The Great Divorce* (New York: HarperOne, 2001).
68 Peter Schakel, "Heaven and Hell as Idea and Image in C.S. Lewis," C.S. Lewis, May 7, 2010, https://www.cslewis.com/heaven-and-hell-as-idea-and-image-in-c-s-lewis.

The biblical understanding of heaven and eternity is not individualistic and independent; it is not about getting your mansion so that you can watch TV by yourself. It is about God; it is about worship; and it is about being completely known and loved as a part of the best community imaginable where no sin, selfishness, or relational hurt will be experienced ever again. For you see, the problem is not that community is bad. The problem is that, in this life, community is hard; and we are frail. But it will not always be this way.

A Deeper Look at Loneliness

Loneliness is not about being physically alone. One can be in a crowd, in a marriage, or on a team and experience loneliness. Loneliness is primarily about the emotional experience of feeling unseen, unknown, and like no one really cares. It is waking up at 2:00 a.m. terrified from a nightmare and not being able to think of one person you could talk to about it. It is having good news but feeling there is no one to share it with. It is going out with your college buddies but leaving the evening feeling empty and wondering if anyone actually cared about a word you said. It is sitting alone in your apartment on Christmas Day, while all your coworkers post pictures of themselves with their families looking so stinking happy. It is coming "home" to an empty house or a disconnected spouse, whose only response when you try to talk about your day is "Uh huh" and keep scrolling on their phone.

Feeling alone in your physical or emotional suffering (or any emotion) is one of the most terrifying experiences known to man. There is a reason solitary confinement is a form of torture. At our core, we were made for emotional intimacy.

Loneliness can be a season, or loneliness may be a long struggle. Loneliness does not always look the same for everyone. Some experience loneliness because of a physical separation not within their control, and some choose to be alone because of past experiences. I do not attempt to make light of the fact that different people experience different situations, some of which are excruciatingly painful. In a way, relationships are hard work for everyone; and in a way, they are even harder for some.

But whatever the reason or situation one experiences loneliness, the way forward is similar—vulnerability. Ah, there is that word again. We have been here before. If we are serious about not being lonely, no matter how we may have gotten there, we have to be vulnerable. We have to risk being hurt. We have to allow others into our authentic thoughts, feelings, and desires. We cannot be seen, known, and emotionally cared for by others if we do not share with them.

God is an exception to this. As we have mentioned, Psalm 139 gives us a glimpse into truth that our Creator and Father knows our thoughts and the motives of our hearts before we have spoken them. But people are not like that. We are not mind readers. And many of us are too busy, distracted, and preoccupied with maintaining our own image that we will not even try to emotionally read a person who seems fine on the outside.

A Word to Men

Men in particular can find emotional intimacy a challenge. It is partly due to Western concepts of masculinity. There is a societal message that men are supposed to be emotionally independent, that they do not have emotional needs, and that they are supposed to manage their feelings without sharing them with anyone. We tell little boys not to cry or be so sensitive, to be emotionally tough, and to be in control of their emotions; and we model that the only acceptable masculine emotion is anger or confidence.

But let us look to Jesus, not Tony Stark. Jesus modeled vulnerability. We see Him weeping at the death of His friend and the emotional suffering of others who loved Lazarus; we see Him moved with compassion for the hurting, asking for company from His friends, asking the Father to consider making it easier, and expressing a feeling of abandonment.[69]

Acknowledge your need for friendship. Accept that a relational need for other people is not feminine, a sign of weakness, or a character flaw. When Jesus was in the garden right before He was led to a torturous death, He told his friends, "'My soul is very sorrowful, even to death; remain here, and watch with me.' And going a little farther He fell on His face and prayed, saying, 'My Father, if it be possible, let this cup pass from me; nevertheless, not as I will, but as you will.' And He came to the disciples and found them sleeping. And He said to Peter, 'So, could you not watch with me one hour?'"[70]

In Luke's account, we read that an angel came to Jesus in the garden to comfort Him, as His friends were too sleepy to stay up.[71] I find it interesting that even though His friends failed Him, He still asked for their help. He modeled vulnerability and need for others, even though they failed Him.

---

69   John 11:33-38; Matthew 9:36; Matthew 26:36-38; Matthew 26:39; Mark 15:34
70   Matthew 26:38-40
71   Luke 22:41-45

Let others know that you are looking for community and friendship. While working on this book, my husband shared an experience with me that led him to find friendship in an unusual way. At the end of a series that my husband's men's Bible study group was going through, the leader asked what everyone appreciated from the study. Several people said they appreciated the new information and gaining a fresh perspective. But one man admitted he was just there for the fellowship. My husband was impressed by his courage and vulnerability to acknowledge that he was seeking community. This encouraged my husband to ask him to lunch, and the man said yes.

Because our culture is so busy and distracted, everyone assumes everyone else is uninterested in developing a friendship. Sometimes, simply letting others know that you are open to spending time together opens the door. Relationships are hard work, but it is important work.

If we are serious about building a strong community, we must let go of our control, pride, unrealistic expectations, and laziness. Relationships with other humans are messy and challenging, and there is often much that is out of our control. We must put people in their proper perspective. Jennie Allen, in her book *Find Your People*, summarizes it like this: "You will disappoint me. I will disappoint you. God will never disappoint us."[72] We need God's grace to go on the journey of truly loving imperfect people.

"He who loves his dreams of community more that the Christian community itself becomes a destroyer of the latter."[73]You can do this. We need you to do this—not just for yourself (because that matters) but

---

72   Jennie Allen, *Find Your People: Building Deep Community in a Lonely World* (Carol Stream, IL: WaterBrook, 2022), 43.

73   Dietrich Bonhoffer, *Life Together: The Classic Exploration of Christian Community* (New York: HarperOne, 1954).

also because there are other people who need you to be their community. One of the reasons so many people, especially young people, are going to professional counseling is because they lack community. I am not saying it's the only reason, of course, or that you will never need to see a professional if you have community. I am saying that a good therapist offers what our culture is so desperately looking for.

Think about it: a good therapy session is slow. The therapist has set aside time just for you. Good therapy is undistracted. There are no screens, notifications going off, or flashing lights. A good therapy session will reduce your need to maintain a perfect image. One is invited to be authentic, vulnerable, and understood. And finally, good therapy curbs loneliness (albeit temporarily). We feel validated, connected, and relatable in our human experience. What is crazy is that in our culture, paying a professional can feel like the only way we can get these needs met. And that is assuming you can find a good therapist who is aware of modern mental health dangers and is actively protecting against them themselves. What if we made a commitment to be this kind of friend, spouse, or church member to the people in our lives?

COMMON OBJECTIONS

Why put so much energy into building relationships with people when they just end, anyway? Relationships are sticky and messy, and "ain't nobody got time for that." Even if you do not have a fall-out with someone, people move away or move on for one reason or another. What is the point?

The point is, Jesus told us to not stop meeting together; to spur one another on.[74] We must make the effort because Jesus left us an example

---

here on earth about how to fellowship with regular people who do stupid and annoying things. And guess what, you are annoying, too, at times! And don't you want people to not give up on you?

Yes, people move on. I have had the immense blessing of some super sweet fellowship seasons in my life. I really bonded with some of my colleagues in graduate school. Graduate school was tough; and there was a group of us that studied together, discussed ideas, worked on group projects, interned together, and even traveled overseas together. Some of these friends would come to my house for "Souplication," our name for a time of homemade soup and prayer (permission to laugh here at our corny name). Many of us were away from our home areas, and we became a kind of family for each other.

I do not get to fellowship with that group in person anymore. That season is done. In some ways, it is a kind of grief. I miss that which is no longer here. But that does not mean it was not worth it. That does not mean that I cannot enjoy other seasons of fellowship in my life. Sometimes, we need to let go of the "good, ol' days" standard if it keeps us from missing out on the season that we are in right now. Also, be encouraged that if those people you miss are followers of Jesus, you will see them again. We will have all of eternity to catch up with dear brothers and sisters in the best reunion ever. Personally, I cannot wait. In the meantime, let's look at some ways we can address loneliness.

LEARN TO RECOGNIZE WHAT YOU NEED

All humans have emotional and relational needs. We can get these needs met through what author John Townsend calls "relational nutrients." In his book, *People Fuel,* Townsend lays out twenty-two relational nutrients that people need to be emotionally healthy. Examples include affirmation, validation, comfort, insight, celebration, and advice. He points out that we can get these nutrients from a variety of people and that no one relationship is sufficient.[75] Remember, people will disappoint us; so we need a community, a support system (as opposed to one support person), throughout the course of our lives. No one person can provide all of our relational nutrients. It is up to each of us to first understand which nutrients we need at a given time and express that need to trusted people—not perfect people, but trusted people around us. I know it may sound harsh or frustrating, but the truth is that people often do not know what you need if you do not know it yourself and ask them for it. If you do not ask for it, you may be waiting a long time.

PRACTICE SOLITUDE

What? Isn't this chapter about community and spending time with other people? One of the largest changes to our modern world is a lack of true solitude. Cal Newport, in *Digital Minimalism,* highlights the significant solitude deprivation of our time. He points out that because of cell phones and the internet, we are often not truly alone with our own thoughts.[76] Our minds are filled with other people's thoughts through social media posts, advertisements, podcasts, images, films, and the like. Many people, especially young people, are rarely alone with their own thoughts; or if they are, they are very uncomfortable with it. They are distressed by the experience; therefore, they will distract and decide solitude is unpleasant.

---

75   John Townsend, *People Fuel: How Energy from Relationships Form Life, Love, and Leadership* (Grand Rapids, MI: Zondervan, 2019).

76   Cal Newport, *Digital Minimalism: Choosing a Focused Life in a Noisy World* (New York: Penguin Random House, 2019).

Solitude is a precious gift to our brains and souls. It allows our minds to slow down and process what is happening within us. It allows us space to make sense of our environment and to reflect on our decisions, our needs, our relationships, our dreams, and our desires. This is a crucial step to being able to do what we mentioned in the previous paragraphs. We cannot be vulnerable and authentic with other humans if we do not allow time to be vulnerable and authentic with ourselves. How can we know what we want or need if we do not take the time to ponder our inner thought life? We cannot.

Solitude also allows us time to commune with God. Quiet time alone with God is a tradition practiced by followers of Yahweh since ancient times. No mere mortal can fulfill our deepest needs and desires. God is always available, undistracted, and uninterested in pretense or show. He is completely secure, always faithful, and totally committed to our health and well-being from before we were conceived in the womb and for an eternal future.[77]

Protect Against Modern Dangers of Hurriedness and Overstimulation

This cannot be stressed enough. One of the main things people tell me is keeping them from building community is busyness. Relationships take work and time, and many of us are simply too busy. We have not prioritized intimate relationships. I agree with John Mark Comer that "love is painfully time consuming," but what else matters more?[78] If we do not have time for love, what are we doing? Hurriedness

---

77   Jeremiah 1:5; 1 Thessalonians 4:17
78   John Mark Comer, *The Ruthless Elimination of Hurry* (Colorado Springs: Water-Brook, 2019).

keeps us stressed, irritable, and lonely; and it is worth fighting against. The cost of giving in is too high.

PRIORITIZE IN-PERSON RELATIONSHIPS AND REDUCE ONLINE RELATIONSHIPS

There is this strong cultural belief that social media relationships are valuable. Maybe for some, they do have some value; but for me, the little relational connection I may gain through online communication is not enough to justify how much it takes from my mental and emotional space and therefore takes from in-person relationships. For me, it is no longer worth it. I want to put my time and attention on meaningful, in-person interactions. I cannot afford to do otherwise. My soul craves emotionally intimate relationships.

> The idea that it's valuable to maintain vast numbers of weak-tie social connections is largely an invention of the past decade or so . . . humans have maintained rich and fulfilling social lives for our entire history without needing the ability to send a few bits of information each month to people we knew briefly during high school. The small boosts you receive from posting on a friend's wall or liking their latest Instagram photo can't come close to compensating for the large loss experienced by no longer spending real world time with that same friend.[79]

Research has shown—and deep down, we know—that online social interactions are not as good for us as meaningful, in-person

---

79   Cal Newport, *Digital Minimalism: Choosing a Focused Life in a Noisy World* (New York: Penguin Random House, 2019), 141, 155.

relationships; but so many, especially our young people, are surviving off of short texts, emojis, and thumbs ups; and the result is relational starvation—an epidemic of loneliness. We cannot replace relationships with real people with a relationship with a computer. Jean Twenge, an academic who studies cross-generational differences, reports that one of her research studies shows: "The results could not be clearer: teens who spend more time on screen activities . . . are more likely to be unhappy, and those who spend more time on nonscreen activities . . . are more likely to be happy. There's not a single exception."[80]

Twenge goes on to report that those with heavy online or social media use are more likely to be depressed, experience cyber bullying, and report loneliness. I love her advice in light of this information: "Do not sleep with it [your phone] or give it nude pictures of yourself. It is not your lover. Do not continuously turn your attention to it when you are talking to someone in person. It is not your best friend."[81]

Changing our relationship with media will be hard at first, but I strongly invite you to consider reducing social media if you experience anxiety, depression, anger, or loneliness. We end this point with one more quote from Cal Newport: "Because digital minimalists spend so much less time connected to their peers [online], it's easy to think of this lifestyle as extreme, but the minimalist would argue that this perception is backward: what's extreme is how much time everyone else spends staring at their screens."[82]

---

80 Jean Twenge, *iGen. Why Today's Super Connected Kids Are Growing Up Less Rebellious, More Tolerant, Less Happy, and Completely Unprepared for Adulthood* (New York: Atria Books, 2018), 77.

81 Jean Twenge, *iGen. Why Today's Super Connected Kids Are Growing Up Less Rebellious, More Tolerant, Less Happy, and Completely Unprepared for Adulthood* (New York: Atria Books, 2018), 77.

82 Cal Newport, *Digital Minimalism: Choosing a Focused Life in a Noisy World* (New York: Penguin Random House, 2019), xv.

TAKE PRESSURE OFF YOURSELF TO HAVE THE "PERFECT COMMUNITY"

You do not have to become a social butterfly if you are not one; you don't have to join five new groups this month; you don't have to find a "bestie" because that's what you see other people doing. Be realistic about what kind of relationships you need in this season of your life. You do not need tons of people. You need a handful of people that you are investing in and allowing them to invest in you. Enjoy the journey. Relationships are hard work, but they do not have to be torture. Loneliness is torture; but building relationships can be exciting!

ASK YOURSELF: WHO IS ALREADY IN MY LIFE?

Who are the people you interact with (in person) on a regular basis? Stop and think through a typical week. What is your routine? Do you go to work or school, care for children, walk your dog, or go to the coffee shop? (Note: Some of you struggle with being too busy and might need to eliminate some things in your routine. Some of you need to add practices to your routine if it mostly consists of online activities by yourself.)

Identify some of the people you could interact with as you go about your weekly routine. Is there a coworker or colleague you could get to know better? Are there other young parents or a single adult who you could invite over for informal play dates with your kids? Are there neighbors who walk their dog or are outside their homes often? Could you slow down and invite someone to join you for coffee consistently on Saturday mornings or whenever you typically go there? Those people are prime opportunities for building community because of the proximity (they are physically close to you and therefore in-person interactions) and because of frequency (relationships take time, so we have to spend consistent time with people in order to feel close to them).

Ask Yourself: Who Is Reaching Out to Me?

I will admit I have spent a lot of time moaning about how hard it is to find friends; and when I do find someone I want to be friends with, they don't seem as interested in me. I had in my head this picture of *my* kind of friend—she is funny and witty and super intelligent and confident. She has great style, but not snobby style—just effortlessly stylish. Oh, and did I mention funny? Basically, I wanted to be friends with Beth from *This Is Us* (anybody else?). But besides the obvious problem that this perfect person I imagined (who, by the way, never did anything wrong and always showed up for me) did not exist, I was missing out on the wonderful (albeit less Beth-like) people in my life. This is foolish, immature, and a consumerist mindset (more on that soon).

So who is reaching out to you? What family members, coworkers, elderly church ladies, awkward teenagers, or quirky neighbors have expressed interest in spending time with you? I know I am not alone in my wishing for an ideal friend fantasy because I hear other people talk about it, too—how hard it is to find friends, how nobody likes them. But what they really mean is "nobody who's my ideal kind of friend is seeking me out."

When I start to ask who *is* seeking them out, often (not always, but often) people will start to think of someone. "Well, my small group leader has mentioned he'd love to get lunch with me, but I just haven't taken him up on it yet." Loneliness can be helped by imperfect people. Ask God to show you the people He has already placed in your life who you could encourage or be encouraged by.

Disclaimer here: I am *not* saying that you should say yes to people who you know are not good for you or you for them. No need to say yes to your ex-boyfriend, your college roommate who was a bad influence, or someone else's wife who you are attracted to. You get the idea. Also, if you currently have a relationship that you know or highly suspect is unhealthy, consider getting some counsel about this relationship. Seek out a respected family member, mentor, or professional counselor and ask the Lord if this is a relationship you need to keep investing in. Sometimes, respectfully parting ways is the wisest and godliest choice.

Be Aware of People in Need in your Local Area and Respond

I think it is crazy and sad that new American parents often feel isolated and alone in the exhausting, monotonous days with little ones. They may get a free meal or two; but for the most part, many are on their own. New parents in past eras (and still in many non-Western cultures) care for new mothers diligently—providing consistent meals, babysitting for older children, being available to talk, or offering practical help and advice. In our culture, many new parents feel they must Google whatever they need to know, instead of asking for help from people in their real life.

There are likely other people in need in your area. Do you know someone who is sick or injured? An elderly or single adult who is alone for a holiday? We assume they must be fine, but I can assure you that many are not fine. Keep asking and keep offering to help in small, practical ways. The little things are actually the big things—the things that matter the most.

STOP "SHOPPING" FOR FRIENDS

We live in a very consumeristic culture. I have said that before in this book, but it is worth repeating. If we want something, we can have it delivered to our door in less than twenty-four hours. This mindset has affected many people's attitudes toward friendships and community. We "shop" for friends, partners, and churches like we shop for a pair of pants. But this was not always the case. In past eras, and still in other parts of the world, you were emotionally close to the people right around you. In a way, they were chosen for us.

Because many of us now move a lot and have the internet, we have access to many more people than we previously had. This can make some of us anxious to find the perfect people. If we see friendships as something we need to research and purchase, it will not work the same. You will find yourself wanting to return it in the drop box at a nearby department store.

BE A PERSON THAT YOU YOURSELF WOULD WANT FOR A FRIEND

I have witnessed people treating their friends like products; and as you can imagine, this is very hurtful. They say sure to a friend's invitation to get lunch at a pizza joint; but in the back of their minds, they are waiting to see if a better offer comes from someone else whose Instagram following is better. There is a lack of commitment that is considered normal in our culture. And this makes building community and reducing loneliness very difficult.

In her book, *Living into Community: Cultivating Practices That Sustain Us*, Christine Pohl says that healthy community members make and keep promises.[83] Of course, there will always be things that come up and prevent us from a well-intended commitment like a blown tire or a sick child; but bailing out on people consistently because you are tired (because you booked yourself too tight or you've been scrolling for an hour) is hurtful and harmful. You may not completely lose the relationship, but you are chipping away at an opportunity to build trust and show that you prioritize that person.

GAIN AN UNDERSTANDING AND PRACTICE HEALTHY BOUNDARIES

One of the reasons many people are hesitant to be in community is because interacting with others can be hard. Maybe some have been hurt by others, taken advantage of, or mistreated in some way. The word *boundaries* can scare some people because it is often a misunderstood idea. Healthy relational boundaries are *not* about putting up emotional walls with other people, ignoring people, being rude, or isolating yourself so you never have to deal with anyone who annoys you. On the contrary, healthy boundaries are what allow a relationship to continue through conflict, disappointment, or even betrayal because they establish how you will respond to difficulties.

Boundaries involve separating what is in my sphere of responsibility (in my control) and what is not in my sphere of responsibility (not in my control). For example, let us say I have a friend who is the volunteer coordinator for the children's ministry at my church. I know she is busy and is always in need of more volunteers. She asks me every week if I can make brownies for the kids and volunteers after the services.

---

83   Christine D. Pohl, *Living into Community: Cultivating Practices That Sustain Us* (Grand Rapids, MI: Wm. B. Eerdmans Publishing Co., 2012).

Every week, I dread seeing her because I know she is going to ask me for something; and I am feeling so burned out. I have no margin, and I need a break. But I continue to say yes, even though I know that if I say no, my friend can find someone else to take a turn; and no one will be upset with me. But I keep saying yes and silently begin resenting my friend, even though a plastic smile is on my face.

So who is at fault here? I may be tempted to think that my friend should just see how busy I am and stop asking me to make brownies already! But that is not her sphere of responsibility. It is mine. How is my friend supposed to know that I am feeling burned out? If I continue to say yes and do not express that I need a break, how is she supposed to know? She is in her sphere—making sure the brownies are there. It is my job to know what I need, what I can and cannot do.

Healthy boundaries are also about knowing that it is not my job to read other people's minds. I have personally spent a lot of time and mental energy worrying about what other people were thinking or feeling. Were they mad at me? Were they actually okay with doing the thing I asked them to do? When I practice healthy boundaries, I stop trying to read their minds. If I am really getting signals from them that they are unhappy, I choose authenticity and just ask them, "Hey, are you sure that you can handle that? I may be wrong, but it seems like you are upset about it. It is totally okay if you need a break."

Relationships are so much more enjoyable and beneficial when there are healthy boundaries. And do not wait for others to do it. That is what boundaries are about—being the person God is calling you to be no matter how others act. The *Boundaries* series by Henry Cloud and John Townsend, as well as Lysa Terkeurst's book *Good Boundaries and Goodbyes* are excellent resources in learning this valuable skill.

Practice Good Listening Skills and Show Genuine Interest in Other People

This may be one of the most practical skills in this chapter. In his classic book, *How to Win Friends and Influence People*, Dale Carnegie explains this important life skill. One of the fastest ways to get people to like you is for you to ask about them, show interest in their lives, and be curious about what they do, think, feel, believe, and value. Most people are drawn to and find interesting those who show interest in them.[84] We all long to be known, understood, and found interesting. If you are not in the habit of practicing this, give it a try next time you are interacting with someone. (It helps if your interest is genuine.)

And if you are struggling to find genuine interest in a person, ask God for it. I do not want to just play the game and "win" friends. I long for the heart of Christ, Who demonstrated this way of relating so well. By showing genuine interest in the lives of others, He drew people to Himself. Have fun with this! People are so fascinating, quirky, and strange in their own beautiful ways.

Embrace the Awkward and Utilize Humor

One of the biggest things we fear when it comes to building relationships is embarrassment. This fear holds many people back from taking even minor social risks. But the truth is, few things are as liberating as embracing awkward situations. No one ever died of embarrassment! Fear and shame—yes, those are more serious experiences; but embarrassment, no. So what if you stumble on your words a little or do not know everything about a topic? Be vulnerable

---

84   Dale Carnegie, *How to Win Friends and Influence People* (New Delhi: Srishti Publishers & Distributors, 2020).

and say how you are feeling in the moment. Learn to laugh at yourself. When we let go of needing to maintain a certain image or reputation, it frees us to be authentic and awkward.

This combo is actually gold for building relationships. Think about it. Who were your closest friends growing up? Weren't they the ones you could be yourself around? Your awkward, imperfect self? Yes!

Humor is one of life's greatest gifts. Laughter is good for the body and good for the soul. It has helped humans survive throughout the generations. It brings people together. Humor disarms people's defenses and puts them at ease. But be advised: get to know someone before using sarcasm or making fun of them. Some people need to know your heart before they can accept your teasing as safe.

PRACTICE APOLOGIZING

All relationships have rough patches because all people are imperfect. If you interact with people, there will be times that you hurt them, and they hurt you. When you hurt someone, something as simple as a genuine apology goes a long way. I'm always amazed, though, at how hard this is for people to do (myself included). I have sat with many clients who express deep regret and guilt over how they treated someone; and when I ask if they have apologized, they say, "No, not really."

Confessing and apologizing are so rare in our culture; we really try to avoid ever having to do it. However, these ancient practices of the faith will take you far. And then here is the really impactful part. Follow that apology with, "Would you please forgive me?" Many people have not grown up seeing their parents, teachers, coaches, or other adults sincerely apologize and ask for forgiveness; so this can feel so uncomfortable, so vulnerable. And it is.

But this is the way of Jesus. "Confess your sins to one another."[85]If "your brother has something against you, leave your gift there before the altar and go. First be reconciled to your brother."[86] You do not need anything from the other person. It does not matter if they accept your apology or not. You focus on what God would have you to do.

EXPRESS GRATITUDE

This is a skill we teach little children, but many of us lose this valuable practice somewhere along the way. We simply forget to thank the people in our lives. And sadly, the ones we neglect to thank the most are those who we are closest to and who we interact with on a regular basis. This is so easy and simple to do, but we often forget how powerful it is. And if you really want to go to Relationship Ninja level 9.5, pay attention to a person's personality and love language. How could you express your gratitude in a way that the receiver would be the most impacted? Is it a heartfelt, look-them-in-the-eye thank you? Is it a handwritten note or thoughtfully worded text? How about a small gift like their favorite snack or offering to do a service for them? Most everyone loves to be thanked and appreciated, especially for mundane, non-glorious work. Don't you?

EXPRESS YOUR NEEDS AND ACCEPT HELP FROM OTHERS

When I was a new mom, I felt so overwhelmed all the time. I was embarrassed that other moms seemed to be holding it all together, and I felt like I was barely functioning. Someone told me this valuable advice:

---

85   James 5:16
86   Matthew 5:23-24

Ask for help! And then keep asking for help. And if someone offers to help you, say yes. Of course, there are times when saying yes would not have been a good idea; but the point is that, much of the time, accepting help is a good thing. We can tend to be so independent as Americans. We are like frustrated toddlers trying to carry all of our stuffed animals to the living room, dropping them in the process and screaming, "I can do it myself!" when someone offers to help.

Sure, there are times when we do need to do things ourselves; but as a general rule, I think that Americans sway on the side of too independent. Admitting our vulnerability and asking for help is hard to do; but when we humble ourselves and choose vulnerability, we will find friends. We will find other people want to be helpful (especially if they get thanked for it). It is wins all around.

Do Hard Things with Like-minded People

One of the dangers of an affluent culture is that we have more ability to choose an easier life. There is this idea of a "soft life" floating around, especially with young people. While there are certainly things we can do to reduce unnecessary stress (that's kind of the whole point of this book), the goal is not simply to make our lives easy. As followers of Jesus, we are called to do hard things. We have missions that give us a sense of purpose and that we are part of something bigger than ourselves. If the goal is simply to make your life as cushy as possible, that—in my opinion—is kind of bleak and depressing.

Everyone wants a "bestie," someone who will always be there for them; but if you never engage in difficult tasks with other people, then you will not have the privilege of bonding with another person on a deep meaningful level. On the other hand, shared mission is what brings people together. Some of my deepest, most meaningful connections were with people I did hard things with.

I worked at a wilderness camp for about four years, and that group of counselors—we had a bond. Shared experiences such as living outside year round, going on three-week canoe trips, and leading teens struggling with behavioral issues was a unique experience. We swapped stories, cooked food for each other, sang and played instruments around campfires, went hiking, slid down waterfalls, and prayed for each other. My years at camp were some of the hardest of my life; but strangely, they were also some of the sweetest. I absolutely cherished the camaraderie and the sense of closeness I felt with that group.

You can experience this kind of closeness, too, but you have to put yourself in situations that will challenge you. Maybe it is a mission trip to a foreign country; maybe it's a weekly ministry for inner city children; maybe it's being intentional about caring for lonely or depressed people in your church. Ask God what He may be calling you to, find others with that same calling, and do hard things with other people.

Join a Group and Commit to It for a Certain Amount of Time

It could be a Bible study or men's fitness group. It could be a regular play date group for small children. Circling back to the previous point, volunteering with a group of people is a fantastic way to build connections to your community and strengthen your mental health. There are endless ways to serve in your area. Think of what you are passionate about (and are tempted to vent about on social media), such as animal rights, care for the environment, immigrants' rights, foster care, etc. and actually do something about that issue in your real world by volunteering.

FIND PRACTICAL WAYS TO REMIND YOURSELF OF THE RELATIONSHIPS YOU ARE CURRENTLY CHOOSING TO PRIORITIZE AND INVEST IN

Write reminders on your calendar to check in with people. You could "pin" text threads to the top of your text messages to those you are trying to get to know. This can help remind you to ask how they are doing, schedule a lunch date, or say a prayer for them. You could schedule regular time in your week when you are available and intentional about spending quality time with people.

REMEMBER THAT BUILDING COMMUNITY OR FRIENDSHIP TAKES TIME

In our microwave, two-day shipping culture, we tend to want things instantly. We want Sam and Frodo-level friendship with as much time and mental energy as it takes to order a new pair of shoes. We say, "I tried going to a small group, but I did not really connect with anyone. I do not think it's for me." Or, "I went out for coffee with her once, but I don't think I'll go again. I am kind of busy, anyway." Friendships and community do not develop instantaneously. They require time, work, mental energy, vulnerability, and commitment.

Some studies have suggested that in order to establish a friendship, you need to have at least eleven meaningful interactions, each at least three hours long over the course of six weeks.[87] One thirty-minute

---

87 Addie Page, "Scientists Warn of a 'Friendship Recession'—I'm a Part of It," *A Different Page* (blog), Medium, February 8, 2023, https://medium.com/modern-marriage/scientists-warn-of-a-friendship-recession-im-part-of-it-38a87a5c27d.

coffee break between running errands every couple of months is not enough to develop any kind of meaningful connection. Neither is randomly texting someone. It takes time. Some believe that especially post COVID-19 pandemic, we have experienced "learned loneliness" as a culture. "A phenomenon where people adjust to isolation. It is not that people do not want to socialize anymore; rather, it is an unfulfilled need that they've learned to live with."[88] If you are serious about fighting loneliness and improving your mental health in this area, you will need to commit to doing the hard work. I believe it is worth it.

REMEMBER PEOPLE WILL NEVER BE ABLE TO FULFILL ALL OF YOUR EMOTIONAL NEEDS

One of my friends, Trina Yoder, put this so well; so I'm just going to quote her:

> You're mainly writing this chapter to those who aren't deeply rooted in community. I think there's another group of people—the people who are lonely despite being rich in community. Those people could be encouraged to pursue intimacy with the Lord. Personally speaking—I am rich in friendships, and I have people I can talk to about hard things; but despite the gold mine of people around me and even though I'm in a good marriage, I still sometimes feel lonely. Sometimes there's a specific situation that I might be facing, but often I think it's simply God giving me an invitation to draw near to Him. There are some places in our hearts that

88   Sanya Nayeem, "How 'learned loneliness' is the reason why we're missing out on friendships," *Gulf News*, March 11, 2023, https://gulfnews.com/amp/games/play/spell-it-how-learned-loneliness-is-the-reason-why-were-missing-out-on-friendships-1.1678290778784.

no amount of connection with humans can fix, and I think God meant it to be that way because He desires to fill us at the place of our deepest need.[89]

All the principles in this book build off one another. As we slow down and reduce distractions, we foster space for authentic relationships. It may seem overwhelming, but we can do this. I believe the church is ready to rise to the challenge. As the church, we can model good mental health and good community. I refuse to be hurried, distracted, preoccupied with proving myself, and disconnected from genuine human connection. Brothers and sisters, our mental and emotional well-being are at stake. May it not be so of the people of God. There are things we can do! Will it be hard at times? Yes, but by the Power that is at work within us, through the Holy Spirit, there is hope. Take courage.

REFLECTIVE QUESTIONS:

1. In what ways do you see loneliness as a problem for our culture?

2. Was there ever a season of loneliness in your life? Are you lonely right now? Who are you closest to?

3. Do you struggle with making friends or feeling connected to community?

4. Was there ever a time when you had a close friend or experienced close community? What was the nature of that time? Why do you think the friendship/community worked?

89   Trina Yoder, email message to author, January 5, 2024.

5. What holds you back from building friendships/ community? What hesitations or objections do you have to doing the hard work of relationships?

6. What is one step you could take to practice engaging in healthy community? Who is one person you could reach out to in the coming weeks?

RECOMMENDED RESOURCES:

- *People Fuel* by John Townsend (Christian perspective)
- *Boundaries* series by Henry Cloud and John Townsend (Christian perspective)
- *Find Your People* by Jennie Allen (Christian perspective)
- *Good Boundaries and Goodbyes* by Lysa Terkeurst (Christian perspective)

CHAPTER 5

Two Vitamins for the Soul

"While other people are complaining about how busy they are,
you will just be smiling sympathetically, unable to relate. While other
people are living a life of stress and chaos, you will be living a life of
impact and fulfillment . . . an act of quiet revolution."[90]

—Greg McKeown

In this book, we have focused on looking at modern dangers to our mental health; but let us also consider two "vitamins" for your soul—universally good practices for our mental health—that cross generational, socio-economic, and ethnic backgrounds.

VITAMIN 1: TIME IN NATURE

Consider this quote by Abraham Lincoln: "I can see how it might be possible for a man to look down upon the earth and be an atheist, but I cannot conceive how a man could look up into the heavens and say there is no God."[91]

---

90 Greg McKeown, *Essentialism: The Disciplined Pursuit of Less* (New York, NY: Crown Business, 2014).
91 Dr. Ed Young, "The Winning Walk Devotional Listen Carefully,"February 5th, 2021. https://winningwalk.org/read/devotionals/listen-carefully-2021.

Since the beginning of time, man has looked with wonder on creation and nature. But in our modern world, it is possible for many of us to go an entire day without spending time outside. We go from the house, to the car, to the office, to the car, to the restaurant, to our kid's dentist appointment, and back home again . . . to the TV or phone. If we do go outside, we are often busy and distracted—think football game—with a lot of people, noise, and comparison. That is not the kind of therapeutic time in nature I am talking about. So my question for you is how much time do you spend in nature on a weekly basis—walking, sitting, listening, breathing, discovering, feeling, or just being?

Researchers have found links between time in nature and improved "cognitive function, brain activity, blood pressure, and sleep."[92] Studies have also shown time in nature to reduce mental illnesses, such as anxiety and depression.[93]

Why is time in nature therapeutic? I suggest a few reasons here.

Time in nature puts life into the right perspective.

I invite you to consider the following verses. Go slowly. Read the words out loud if you can.

- "For the Lord is a great God, and a great King above all gods. In his hand are the depths of the earth; the heights of the mountains are His also. The sea is His, for He made it, and

92   Marcia P. Jimenez, et al. "Associations between Nature Exposure and Health: A Review of the Evidence." *International Journal of Environmental Research and Public Health* vol. 18,9 4790, April 30, 2021, https://doi.org/10.3390/ijerph18094790.
93   Kirsten Weir, "Nurtured by Nature," American Psychological Association, April 20, 2020, https://www.apa.org/monitor/2020/04/nurtured-nature.

His hands formed the dry land. Oh come, let us worship and bow down; let us kneel before the Lord, our Maker! For He is our God, and we are the people of His pasture, and the sheep of His hand" (Psalm 95:3-7).

- "But ask the beasts, and they will teach you; the birds of the heavens, and they will tell you; or the bushes of the earth, and they will teach you; and the fish of the sea will declare to you. Who among all these does not know that the hand of the Lord has done this? In His hand is the life of every living thing and the breath of all mankind" (Job 12:7-10).

- "Hear this, oh Job; stop and consider the wondrous works of God. Do you know how God lays his command upon them and causes the lightening of his cloud to shine? Do you know the balancings of the clouds, the wondrous works of him who is perfect in knowledge" (Job 37:14-16).

- "When I look at Your heavens, the work of Your fingers, the moon and the stars, which You have set in place, what is man that You are mindful of him, and the son of man that You care for him?" (Psalm 8:3-4).

Time in nature reminds us Who God is: His glory; His power; His creativity; and His utter and complete control over all people, nations, times, thoughts, feelings, intentions, ideas—both good and evil—He is sovereign over all. Whatever it is that you are wrestling with, it does not surprise Him. It does not confuse Him. It does not thwart His plans and purpose.

Time in nature reminds us that we are created beings—small, limited, imperfect, fallible, finite, fearful, and out of control. And it reminds us who we are: eternally loved, chosen, elevated above creation, individually unique, reflective of God's image, noticed, and tended to like a vulnerable lamb.

It reminds us that we are not in control. There are so many plants, animals, fungi, minerals, and weather patterns that are sustained without us evening knowing they exist. God is working out a grand story that is so much bigger and more epic than we could imagine. He is taking care of all of it, and we get to be a tiny, little piece. We are so small and yet so significant at the same time.

When we worry about how our car will get fixed, how our bills will get paid, how our kids will make it in college, how our health will stand up, or anything else humans concern themselves with, time in nature can remind us that there is much that is not in our control. And this is a good thing.

The seasons in nature remind us that there are seasons of life as well. This, too, shall pass. "For everything there is a season, and a time for every matter under heaven."[94] The difficult things we go through will pass, and new challenges and joys will come. And in the end, a new season will begin—an eternity of purpose, belonging, and joy.

Time in nature is grounding.

One effective tool in reducing anxiety is grounding techniques. Most of what we are upset about is in the past or the future. Grounding exercises bring attention and awareness to the present moment, right where you are. Grounding exercises include becoming aware of your five senses—sight, smell, hearing, touch, and taste—and

---

94 Ecclesiastes 3:1

therefore, becoming more present to where you actually are in that moment. Intentional time in nature is very grounding. There are so many things to see, hear, touch, smell, and even taste. Tuning into the sensations around you can be extremely comforting and calming. As we have discussed, our modern life often includes too much stimulation, noise, and lights that excite and arouse. Nature arouses in all the right ways.

Time in nature is slow.

We have spent a whole chapter in this book exploring the mental health benefits of slowing down, and nature does this organically. If you have ever spent an overnight trip hiking or camping in the wilderness, you know what I mean. Time seems to stop in some ways. You can feel the stresses and expectations melt away as you watch the sun rise in a blast of color, as you listen to the songbirds composing the most beautiful piece of music, and as you feel the cool autumn breeze gently blow your hair. It is downright good for the soul.

Time in nature is an equalizer.

In nature, no one is better than another. Whether your net worth is fifteen million or fifteen cents, the rose smells just as sweet; the birds still sing for you; and the fire ants still bite you. Nature does not discriminate its beauties or its treasures. They are for all. You are enough—good-looking enough, wealthy enough, smart enough, brave enough, talented enough, and privileged enough for your soul to be soothed by this free and readily available gift on this beautiful blue gem we call Earth.

Finally, nature is beautiful.

The sun rises on a cold, late November morning. The skies are cotton-candy pink and blue. Rays of soft sunlight stream through almost-barren branches. The air is cool and crisp and smells deliciously of pine and morning dew. As the bright light of our solar system's star rises, the sky changes. The colors grow warmer, and the clouds change shape: first a bird, now a bear, now a bee. It is as if the landscape is an art gallery and the sky a magnificent piece—an evolving, unfolding canvas that is different one moment to the next. The work of a great Artist, the Artist above all artists, is dabbling in His brushes this morning—a most exquisite living, moving, breathing masterpiece. And this just one of His works.

From the intricacies of a spider's web to the majesty of a roaring cascade, nature is beautiful. It is not always practical, but it is invaluable. It is *extra*. It is extravagant. God could have chosen to make our world colorless and drab, but He did not. Nature's beauty is a gift from the Creator to us, His children. Nature's beauty brings us joy; it sooths and calms us. It causes us to weep from the sheer glory of it if we take the time to enjoy it—to drink it in, to be thankful, and to be loved upon in this way.

Some people may object to spending time in nature, saying it is too hot or too cold, too polluted, or too crowded in the city where they live. I hear you. I have had seasons in my life where quality time in nature seemed difficult to come by. During one particular season, when I was in a large foreign city, I longed for some private quiet time outdoors. But it was too dangerous to go anywhere by myself. But the Lord was very kind to me in that I discovered that right outside my second story window, there was an odd little ledge—not a porch, mind you—but just a little ledge big enough for maybe a potted plant or two that I could squeeze out onto. I would go out in the evening before bed when it was dark and look up at the few brave stars that strained their lights just enough for me to see them through the city skies. It was not exactly a *National Geographic*-sponsored tour; but it was humbling, reminding, grounding, slow, non-judgmental, and soothing.

Unless you spend your life locked up in a windowless prison cell, you have the opportunity to enjoy this wondrous freely accessible gift from God. Overnight wilderness camping may not be for you. That is fine. Find time and ways to slow down; pause even for just a few seconds; and observe the sights, sounds, and sensations of the natural world. Open your window if you can. Pause before opening the door to your office building. Take your time walking from your car to your home. Eat your lunch outside sitting on a step, log, or truck bed. Open a window nearby and listen to the crickets. Embrace opportunities to invite God and His wondrous creation into that moment. More times than not, you will be glad that you did.

Vitamin 2: Gratitude

"Do not be anxious about anything, but in everything by prayer and supplication with thanksgiving let your requests be made known to God. And the peace of God, which surpasses all understanding, will guard your hearts and your minds in Christ Jesus"(Phil. 4:6-7).

Gratitude is something that every major religion (Islam, Judaism, Christianity, Hinduism, and Buddhism) recognizes as important to healthy spiritual existence. Secular science has recognized the power of gratitude as well. Bringing to mind the people and things we are grateful for increases dopamine and serotonin in the brain. These chemicals contribute to feelings of happiness and are key ingredients in psychotropic medications that attempt to regulate and improve mood. Expressing gratitude strengthens the immune system, decreases stress hormones, and relaxes the muscles in the body.[95]

Dan Siegel, in his book *Aware,* describes how mindfulness (the practice of being aware) can greatly affect our minds and bodies. He uses an analogy of a teaspoon of salt. The salt represents our unpleasant thoughts, emotions, and experiences. If you put a teaspoon of salt into a shot glass amount of water and swallow it down, the experience will be quite unpleasant. You will definitely taste the salt and feel its impact. You will feel it burn and be left with the taste in your mouth. But if you put that same teaspoon of salt into a one-and-a-half-gallon pitcher of water and swallow, it will be a completely different experience. You may still notice the saltiness; but its effects will be slight, as the pure drinking water dilutes the salt's potency.[96]

In the same way, when we become aware of other things (people, places, items, thoughts, feelings, and experiences) in our lives, we do not take away the hard things. A teaspoon is still a teaspoon. We do not deny that the teaspoon of salt is unpleasant to drink. However, mindfulness brings awareness to all the other things that are going on in our lives, including things we like. Gratitude is not just a "think more positively" approach. Gratitude is not lying. It is not denying the situation or our feelings in it. It is not saying you're fine if you're really

---

95   Robert Emmons, *Gratitude Works: A 21-Day Program for Creating Emotional Prosperity* (San Francisco, CA: Jossey-Bass, 2013).

96   Daniel Siegel, *Aware: The Science and Practice of Presence* (New York: Penguin Random House, 2018).

feeling devastated. Instead, recognizing what you are grateful for is actually about being more truthful.

One of my definitions of mental illness is a pattern of seeing things differently than they really are. For example, anxiety overestimates the threat and underestimates your abilities to manage it. Depression causes one to see probabilities as always against them and that things will never change. Psychotic disorders, such as bipolar mania and schizophrenia, are characterized by distortions of reality in people's thoughts. Gratitude is not living in disillusionment but truth.

Gratitude is a weapon. There is supernatural power in practicing gratitude. When we choose to acknowledge God's gifts to us, we wage spiritual warfare. We push back against strongholds of despair, depression, and discouragement. We say, "No, not today, Satan." We join Job in declaring, "Though He [God] slay me, I will hope in Him."[97] We join David in proclaiming, "The Lord is my strength and my shield; in Him my heart trusts, and I am helped; my heart exults, and with my song I give thanks to Him."[98]

I believe something happens in the spiritual realm when we choose to obey God with our gratitude, especially when it's hard and the world would say give up and give into despair. Gratitude also just works. In moments of fear; panic; or intrusive thoughts, disciplining the mind to focus on that which we have to be grateful for calms the body and the spirit.

There are countless stories of people around the world, throughout thousands of years, who have gone through horrendous suffering, tragedy, injustice, and loss. One of the timeless tools that humans

---

97   Job 13:15
98   Psalm 28:7

have utilized is gratitude. They chose to bring to awareness that which they did have or what was going well. In her famous book, *The Hiding Place,* Corrie ten Boom tells a story of her time in Ravensbrück concentration camp in 1944. Conditions were horrible in so many ways, not least of which was that the barracks were infested with fleas. Corrie's sister, Betsie, insisted that they should be grateful in all things; but Corrie was angry. There was nothing to be thankful for when it came to the fleas.

A little while later, they overheard that the reason the guards had not raided their barracks recently was because the fleas were so bad. The guards were repelled from going in there. This allowed Corrie and the other followers of Jesus to study the Bible, pray, and worship together during those extremely difficult days. So in a way, they became grateful for the fleas.[99] There are many other stories of Christians and non-Christians alike who have found strength in trouble by calling to mind that which they have to be grateful for.

So what else is true about your situation? The thing that is causing you emotional pain? Chances are that 100 percent of your life is not falling apart. Do not ignore the hard things, and do not ignore the wonderful things. What people, foods, animals, sunrise, clouds, sound of water, victorious football game, non-leaking roof, and non-throbbing head do you have to be grateful for today?

REFLECTIVE QUESTIONS:

1.   Do you think time in nature is important?

2.   How much time do you typically spend experiencing nature in a given week?

---

99   Corrie ten Boom, *The Hiding Place* (Ada, MI: Baker Publishing Group, 2023).

3. Do you have a favorite memory of being in nature?

4. What holds you back from spending time in nature?

5. What is one step you could take to spend more intentional time in nature?

6. Do you think gratitude is important?

7. How do you do with expressing gratitude?

8. What are three things you are grateful for right now?

9. What holds you back from acknowledging the things you are grateful for?

10. Is there a routine or practice that could help you practice gratitude?

Conclusion

As you have read and reflected on these modern dangers to mental health, some of you may experience unpleasant emotions such as overwhelm or guilt. If that is the case, thank you for sticking it out. Know that *no one* is perfectly balanced in any of these areas. I have struggled with every one of these dangers. I have written this content because I have struggled with this content. They are cultural dangers no one is immune to, but there is also so much hope.

Hear my word of encouragement to you—neither should you become overwhelmed or paralyzed by all you need to "fix" in your life, nor foster a doomsday mentality that you should bunker down in a hole somewhere and wait until Jesus comes back. This book is meant to inspire and to give courage; it is not a list of rules to measure how good you are doing. It is not a competition, remember?

Some of you may be encouraged and motivated after reading this book. If so, please share this book and what has stood out to you with others. Many aspects of modern culture are counter to God's design, but I have a lot of hope that followers of Jesus can influence the culture for good when we live differently.

Three words come to mind: grace, grace, and grace. We need God's grace over every aspect of our lives—grace to believe in Him, grace to trust Him, and grace for ourselves—not because we deserve it but because

God has already freely given it to those who are His. The Good News of Jesus is that we are not good enough; but Jesus paid for us through His sacrificial death. And by His wounds, we are free. Perfectionism is not possible or necessary. In fact, unrelenting standards and shame toward ourselves and others actually hinders growth and keeps us from living out the calling God has for each of us.

Accept God's grace that your mental health is not (and will not be until the new Heaven and earth) wholly intact. *And* at the same time, be inspired to growth in areas that you can change. Consider the Alcoholics Anonymous' prayer: "That I may be reasonably happy in this life, and supremely happy in the next."[100] Start small if you need to. Choose one practical step to take from each section of the book. Just one step. It does matter. "Greater is He who is in you than He who is in the world."[101] And grace. Remember grace for the journey.

If you have come upon this book and you are not a follower of Jesus, or maybe you assumed you were but you are realizing that you did not understand the true gospel, you are loved. There is an invitation for you to recognize your need for God and allow Him to comfort you—to quite literally save your life. No one is too far gone or too out of reach. Jesus came for you, friend.

"The world is indeed full of peril, and in it there are many dark places,
but still there is much that is fair. And though in all lands,
love is now mingled with grief, it grows perhaps the greater."[102]

—J.R.R. Tolkien

---

100 "The AA Prayer (Serenity Prayer) Explained," Alcoholics Resource Center, September 11, 2023, https://alcoholicsanonymous.com/aa-serenity-prayer.

101 1 John 4:4

102 J.R.R. Tolkien, *The Fellowship of the Ring* (New York: HarperCollins, 2009).

Reflective questions:

1. Which of the modern dangers to our mental health do you think impacts you the most?

2. What stood out to you in this book? Were there any sections or ideas that you had not previous considered?

3. What did you appreciate about this book?

4. Did you disagree with anything in this book?

5. Are there steps you plan to take in light of the material in this book?

6. Do you know anyone who could benefit from this book?

Acknowledgments

I want to thank my husband, Greg, for listening to me talk about this project night upon night and for encouraging me when I had irrational anxiety attacks about citations! I am so grateful to you. Special thanks to the group of people who read drafts of this book and gave me their encouragement and feedback: Greg Bateman, Bethany Kung, Natalie Nolt, Trina Yoder, Jessica Barley, Walter Howard, Mary Campbell Norman, Kent Bateman, Brent Leaders, and Peter Hubbard. I am grateful to Samuel Lowry and the team at Ambassador International, who saw potential in this little book. And of course, I am eternally grateful to the Lord: no words could express.

Bibliography

"AA Prayer (Serenity Prayer) Explained, The." Alcoholics Resource Center. September 11, 2023. https://alcoholicsanonymous.com/aa-serenity-prayer.

Abrams, Zara. "Growing Concerns About Sleep." *American Psychological Association,* June 1, 2021.https://www.apa.org/monitor/2021/06/news-concerns-sleep#:~:text=Since%20the%20pandemic%20began%2C%20researchers,in%20America%20 2021%2C%20APA).

"Adult Data 2023." Mental Health America. Last modified 2024.https://www.mhanational.org/the-state-of-mental-health-in-america/archived-reports.

Allen, Jennie. *Find Your People: Building Deep Community in a Lonely World.* Carol Stream, IL: WaterBrook, 2022.

Anderson, Sam. "How many ads do we really see in a day? Spoiler: It's not 10,000." *The Drum,* May 3, 2023.https://www.thedrum.com/news/2023/05/03/how-many-ads-do-we-really-see-day-spoiler-it-s-not-10000.

Aron, Elaine. *The Highly Sensitive Person: How to Thrive When the World Overwhelms You.* New York: Broadway Books, 1996.

Beuchler, Jessica. "The Loneliness Epidemic Persists: A Post-

Pandemic Look at the State of Loneliness Among U.S. Adults." The Cigna Group. Last updated 2024, https://newsroom.thecignagroup.com/loneliness-epidemic-persists-post-pandemic-look.

Bonhoffer, Dietrich. *Life Together: The Classic Exploration of Christian Community*. New York: HarperOne, 1954.

Brown, Brené. *Daring Greatly: How the Courage to be Vulnerable Transforms the Way We Live, Love, Parent, and Lead*. New York, NY: Gotham Books, 2012.

Carnegie, Dale. *How to Win Friends and Influence People*. New Delhi: Srishti Publishers & Distributors, 2020.

Cloud, Henry and John Townsend. *Boundaries: When to Say Yes, How to Say No, To Take Control of Your Life*. Grand Rapids, MI: Zondervan, 2017.

Comer, John Mark. *The Ruthless Elimination of Hurry*. Colorado Springs: WaterBrook, 2019.

"Dealing with Stress: 12 Proven Strategies for Stress Relief from Stoicism." Daily Stoic: Ancient Wisdom for Everyday Life. Last updated 2021. https://dailystoic.com/stress-relief.

Deanglis, Tori. "Young adults are still lonely, but the rates of loneliness are dropping overall." America Psychological Association. July 1, 2023. https://www.apa.org/monitor/2023/07/young-adults-lonely-pandemic#:~:text=67%25,with%2032%25%20of%20the%20nonlonely.

Dillard, Annie. *The Writing Life*. New York: Harper Perennial, 2013.

Emmons, Robert. *Gratitude Works: A 21-Day Program for Creating Emotional Prosperity*. San Francisco, CA: Jossey-Bass, 2013.

Gračanin, Asmir, et al. "Why crying does and sometimes does not seem to alleviate mood: a quasi-experimental study." *Motivation and Emotion* vol. 39, 6, August 23, 2015. https://doi.org/10.1007/s11031-015-9507-9.

Hagerty, Sara. *Unseen: The Gift of Being Hidden in a World that Loves to Be Noticed*. Grand Rapids, MI: Zondervan, 2017.

"Happy Birthday Joan Proctor." Zoological Society of London, August 4, 2017.https://www.zsl.org/news-and-events/news/happy-birthday-joan-procter.

Honore, Carl. *In Praise of Slowness: Challenging the Cult of Speed*. New York: HarperOne, 2005.

"How Loneliness Can Impact Your Health." Cleveland Clinic, September 30, 2024.https://health.clevelandclinic.org/what-happens-in-your-body-when-youre-lonely.

Jimenez, Marcia P. et al. "Associations between Nature Exposure and Health: A Review of the Evidence." *International Journal of Environmental Research and Public Health*. Vol. 18, 9 4790. April 30, 2021. https://doi.org/10.3390/ijerph18094790.

Kerai, Alex. "Cell Phone Use Statistics: Mornings Are for Notifications." *Reviews.org*. July 21, 2023. https://www.reviews.org/mobile/cell-phone-addiction.

Lewis, C.S. *The Great Divorce*. New York: HarperOne, 2001.

Means, Leslie. *So God Made a Mother*. Carol Stream, Illinois: Tyndale, 2023.

Nayeem, Sanya. "How 'learned loneliness' is the reason why we're missing out on friendships." *Gulf News*. March 11, 2023.https://gulfnews.com/amp/games/play/spell-it-how-learned-loneliness-is-the-reason-why-were-missing-out-on-friendships-1.1678290778784.

Newhouse, Leo. "Is crying good for you?" Harvard Health Publishing. March 1, 2021.https://www.health.harvard.edu/blog/is-crying-good-for-you-2021030122020.

Newport, Cal. *Digital Minimalism: Choosing a Focused Life in a Noisy World*. New York: Penguin Random House, 2019.

Orthlund, Dane. *Gentle & Lowly: The Heart of Christ for Sinners and Sufferers*. Wheaton, IL: Crossway, 2020.

Page, Addie. "Scientists Warn of a 'Friendship Recession'—I'm a Part of It." *A Different Page* (blog). Medium. February 8, 2023.https://medium.com/modern-marriage/scientists-warn-of-a-friendship-recession-im-part-of-it-38a87a5c27d.

Pohl, Christine D. *Living into Community: Cultivating Practices That Sustain Us*. Grand Rapids, MI: Wm. B. Eerdmans Publishing Co., 2012.

Price, Catherine. *How to Break Up with Your Phone: The 30-Day Plan to Take Back Your Life*. New York: Ten Speed Press, 2018.

Schakel, Peter. "Heaven and hell as idea and image in C.S. Lewis." C.S. Lewis. May 7, 2010. https://www.cslewis.com/heaven-and-hell-as-idea-and-image-in-c-s-lewis.

Siegel, Daniel. *Aware: The Science and Practice of Presence*. New York: Penguin Random House, 2018.

"Signal Cycle Lengths." National Association of City Transportation Officials. https://nacto.org/publication/urban-street-design-guide/intersection-design-elements/traffic-signals/signal-cycle-lengths.

"Sleep Health." Centers for Disease Control and Prevention/National Center for Health Statistics. Last reviewed February 23, 2023. https://www.cdc.gov/nchs/fastats/sleep-health.htm.

Ten Boom, Corrie. *The Hiding Place*. Ada, MI: Baker Publishing Group, 2023.

Terkeurst, Lysa. *Good Boundaries & Goodbyes: Loving Others Without Losing the Best of Who You Are*. New York: Nelson Books, 2022.

Tolkien, J.R.R. *The Fellowship of the Ring*. New York: HarperCollins, 2009.

Townsend, John. *People Fuel: How Energy from Relationships Form Life, Love, and Leadership*. Grand Rapids, MI: Zondervan, 2019.

Twenge, Jean. *iGen. Why Today's Super Connected Kids Are Growing Up Less Rebellious, More Tolerant, Less Happy, and Completely Unprepared for Adulthood*. New York: Atria Books, 2018.

Valdez, Patricia. *Joan Proctor, Dragon Doctor: The Woman Who Loved Reptiles*. New York: Random House Children's Books, 2018.

Villarreal, Yvonne. "Read the Stirring Monologue about Womanhood America Ferrera delivers in 'Barbie.'" Los Angeles Times. July 23, 2023. https://www.latimes.com/entertainment-arts/movies/story/2023-07-23/barbie-america-ferrera-monologue.

Walker, Kevin. "Reading the stoics with millennials." Lecture at Westmont College, March 2019. https://www.westmont.edu/sites/default/files/users/user551/Walker_0.pdf.

Weir, Kirsten. "Nurtured by Nature." American Psychological Association. April 20, 2020. https://www.apa.org/monitor/2020/04/nurtured-nature.

Wiking, Meik. *The Little Book of Lykke: Secrets of the World's Happiest People*. New York: Harper Collins, 2017.

About the Author

Amber Bateman is a licensed professional counselor with a background in communications and biblical studies. She has worked in a variety of settings, including a therapeutic wilderness camp, sexual assault response program, university counseling center, and private practice. She is passionate about inspiring hope and courage to live life to the fullest. Amber lives near Greenville, South Carolina, with her husband and two sons. She is a foodie and world traveler and a lover of hot tea, herb gardens, and deep discussions. Amber's website can be found at www.delvementalhealth.com.

MORE FROM AMBASSADOR INTERNATIONAL . . .

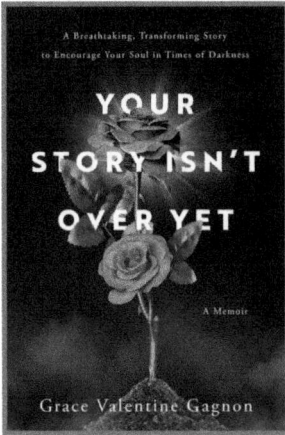

No matter how painful, dark, or challenging your situation is, you can have hope. *Your Story Isn't Over Yet* is a true story of how the sovereignty of God worked through the horrors of domestic violence, sexual assault, abortion, and trauma to ultimately show His unconditional love. Follow Grace's path of pain, loss, and perseverance to a pandemic love story and the joy that can be found only in Jesus.

Day by day this Advent season, as you work your way through Isaiah in *When You Don't Feel Like Celebrating*, keep your heart open to what the Lord has to say. Even if you are struggling to find joy during the holidays, don't turn you away from the source of comfort but instead run to the One Who came to bring light to the darkness of a fallen world.

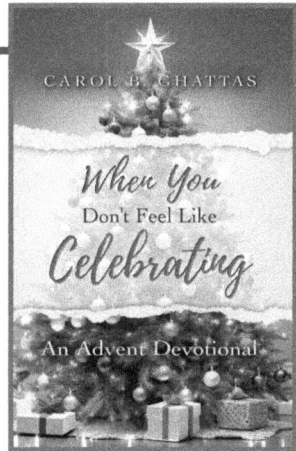

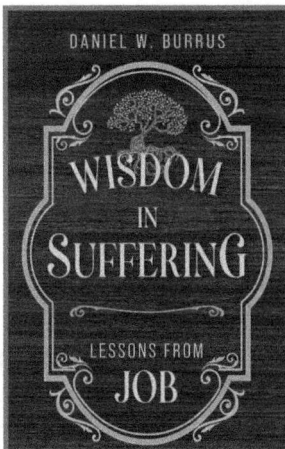

Job is a well-known name, but a deep dive into this portion of God's Word brings truth to light in a way that will illuminate our path when suffering makes life seem dark. Pain and uncertainty do not have to bring us to a place of doubt. Instead, they can be tools in the hands of a wise and loving God to draw us closer to Himself and transform our lives as we learn to trust Him and rely on His wisdom.

www.ingramcontent.com/pod-product-compliance
Lightning Source LLC
Chambersburg PA
CBHW060358090426
42734CB00011B/2171